Fatal Extraction

Mark Carl Rom

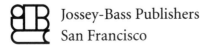 # Fatal Extraction

The Story Behind the Florida Dentist Accused of Infecting His Patients with HIV and Poisoning Public Health

Jossey-Bass Publishers
San Francisco

Copyright © 1997 by Jossey-Bass Inc., Publishers, 350 Sansome Street, San Francisco, California 94104.

Substantial discounts on bulk quantities of Jossey-Bass books are available to corporations, professional associations, and other organizations. For details and discount information, contact the special sales department at Jossey-Bass Inc., Publishers (415) 433–1740; Fax (800) 605–2665.

For sales outside the United States, please contact your local Simon & Schuster International Office.

Jossey-Bass Web address: http://www.josseybass.com

 Manufactured in the United States of America on Lyons Falls Turin Book. This paper is acid-free and 100 percent totally chlorine-free.

Library of Congress Cataloging-in-Publication Data

Rom, Mark C., [date].
Fatal extraction : the story behind the Florida dentist accused of infecting his patients with HIV and poisoning public health / Mark Carl Rom.
     p.   cm.
    Includes bibliographical references and index.
    ISBN 0-7879-0991-2
    1. Acer, David, 1949–1990. 2. Bergalis, Kimberly, 1968–1991—Health. 3. AIDS (Disease)—Patients—Florida—Biography. 4. Dentists—Florida—Biography. 5. Centers for Disease Control (U.S.) 6. Dentists—Malpractice—Florida. 7. Dentist and patient—Florida. I. Title.
RC607.A26A2957 1997
362.1'9697'92—dc21
                                        97-9594
                                         CIP

FIRST EDITION
HB Printing   10 9 8 7 6 5 4 3 2 1

—ᴡᴡ— Contents

Preface

In 1991 the Centers for Disease Control announced that a dentist in Florida had possibly transmitted HIV, the virus that causes AIDS, to a patient while providing her with routine care. The CDC has since reported that the dentist infected five other patients with HIV. These are the first—and thus far the only—cases of a health care worker apparently infecting patients with the deadly virus.

The first patient, a young woman named Kimberly Bergalis, was not prepared to die silently. She lashed out at the public health officials whom she believed had failed to protect her and who seemed not to care. She crusaded for policies that would prevent others from suffering her fate by testing health care workers for HIV, barring infected ones from practicing medicine, or at least requiring those who were infected to disclose this to their patients. Most experts rejected these ideas. The CDC, the agency that announced Bergalis's infection and the same one responsible for advising the medical community on such matters, struggled to resolve the conflict between patients and experts as it developed new policies for health care workers and HIV.

This book focuses on a single dentist, a single patient, a single disease, and a single agency. Yet it is more than a book about the dentist David Acer (rhymes with "hacker"), his patient Kimberly Bergalis, AIDS, and the CDC. The issues it raises concern us all, because we are all patients; we all become ill and seek to become well again; we all ask our government to protect us from life's dangers and uncertainties. Each one of us could be a Kimberly Bergalis when we seek medical care. We all want to know: Will my doctor heal me or harm me? How do I know my doctor is competent, capable—and safe?

These concerns are not just personal, however; ultimately they connect us all to the broader political world in which public health officials work. As patients and citizens, we need to know: What is the government doing to protect us when we obtain medical care? Why is it not doing more?

Many readers might be tempted to answer the first of these two questions with "Not enough" and the second with "Because public health officials are inept, cowardly, or foolish." This book will offer different answers. By showing what the CDC officials (among others) did to resolve the case of the Florida dentist and to make medical settings safer with regard to AIDS, I hope to persuade the reader that the government is doing a lot and that it is not doing other things for good reasons. Still, we have not fully resolved the problem of HIV in medical settings. We thus can and should expect that government, medical providers, and patients will do more to make health care safer and more secure.

The case of the Florida dentist has been a source of unending controversy regarding *who* infected Bergalis and the other patients and *how* the infections occurred. A third question is even more important for our health: *what* should we do to prevent additional infections in the future?

It is my goal, as it was the CDC's, to answer these questions. But to appreciate fully the complexities of this case, we must dig deeper. We need to learn *what* the CDC did to accomplish its tasks, *why* it did these things, and *how* it might have done them better. In this way, perhaps we will come to understand two great mysteries: a medical one about a fatal extraction and a political one about the government's response.

Chapter One introduces the Centers for Disease Control and the main controversies it faced in the case of the fatal extraction. At the time, the CDC was already no stranger to AIDS or to conflict over it; the officials most heavily involved in investigating the fatal extraction had been with the agency since the disease had first appeared. Still, the agency came under enormous scrutiny and criticism for its handling of the case of the Florida dentist. This chapter begins to explore the source of these criticisms and to explain the CDC's behavior.

Chapter Two describes the CDC's attempts to determine how Bergalis contracted HIV. I focus on the CDC's investigators and what they did to collect evidence and also to protect the individuals they investigated. These tasks were not easy. If the government was to determine how Bergalis contracted HIV, its researchers had to collect and confirm highly personal information about her. Few of us, I expect, would be eager to reveal such details about our private lives to bureaucrats, so we have wisely limited the ability of governmental researchers to collect such information. The investigators, moreover, worked in a complex political milieu influenced by the rules and practices of local, state, and federal agencies.

While the second chapter considers whether Bergalis could have been infected by someone other than the dentist, Chapter Three examines whether Dr. Acer did actually transmit HIV to Bergalis and the other patients. Determining whether Acer infected his patients required experiments in molecular biology, where the rules were largely being written as the researchers proceeded. The scientists' work in this pathbreaking study and the uncertainties that they had to resolve provide the focus for this chapter.

But it was not enough for the CDC to investigate *whether* Acer infected the patients; the CDC also needed to learn *how* he did it. Chapter Four considers the main theories—accidental transmission through contaminated dental equipment; direct but accidental contact with Acer's blood (for example, if he nicked his hand while providing treatment); and premeditated murder. We explore here the CDC's efforts to find out which of these theories was correct.

Chapter Five moves away from the CDC's field research to look at the policies and politics of this case. It outlines the reforms advocated by the Bergalis family and patients in general and analyzes them from the perspective of experts in health policy, ethics, and law. It also suggests two strategies that the CDC might take to resolve the conflicts between patients and experts.

Even before the Florida dentist, the CDC had been worried that medical providers could infect their patients. Chapter Six begins by describing the evolution of CDC guidelines regarding health care workers and HIV, then turns to the CDC's efforts to craft policies in light of the Acer case. The CDC was not the only institution with a stake in these policies, however, as numerous groups inside and outside the government pressed their claims on the CDC. Key senators and other high-ranking officials within the Department of Health and Human Services, in particular, used their influence to shape these policies. This chapter concentrates on the political environment surrounding the CDC's public health officials as they attempted to develop guidelines.

Chapter Seven looks outside the CDC to examine what other federal authorities, especially the Occupational Safety and Health Administration (OSHA), the courts, and state governments, were doing to prevent the spread of HIV in medical settings. The CDC, as it turns out, was not the only agency struggling with the policy problems raised by the fatal extraction. Yet no other governmental organization was able to resolve the problems that this case posed any more swiftly and neatly.

The final chapter returns to the critical questions. Did the CDC find the right answers in its investigation and make the best policy choices? How might it work better to create health care settings that are safe and secure?

ACKNOWLEDGMENTS

Many individuals generously contributed their time and talents to this project. They taught me much, although perhaps not as much as they wanted or I needed.

Special thanks go to those who read and commented on part or all of the manuscript while it was a work in progress, especially Ronald Bayer, Chris Foreman, Harold Jaffe, Gerald Myers, Scott Burris, Carol Ciesielski, Mark Barnes, Alan Rocke, Robert Montgomery, Roy Rom, Lisa Rom, and an anonymous reviewer. Robert Montgomery and Steve Sternberg graciously shared their case files with me. David Kirp, Michael Schoenbaum, Richard Scheffler, and Franci Duitch provided advice and encouragement when they were sorely needed. Many people close to this case allowed me to interview them; I thank them. I am certain that others should also be thanked; you know who you are.

My colleagues at Georgetown University and the University of California at Berkeley offered kindness, insights, and humor. George Silberman, Ron Heisterkamp, and Rich Weston at the U.S. General Accounting Office deserve special praise for their contributions. Research assistance was skillfully provided by Nancy Schretzman, Michelle Scheffron, and Ann Cheatham. The Georgetown University Graduate School provided summer research and travel support. Preparation of this volume was also assisted by a grant from The Robert Wood Johnson Foundation, Princeton, New Jersey.

Fellow authors, may I wish you the good fortune of working with the cast at Jossey-Bass. Editors Andrew Pasternack and Barbara Hill had faith in this project when it needed it most. Frank Welsch, Katie Levine, Susan Cho, and others helped turn it into a book; Margaret Sebold, JoAnne Skinner, Lisa Shannon, and Kim Corbin spread the word about it. Matthew Schreiber was helpful in reviewing the manuscript. Nancy Palmer Jones, my copyeditor who favors understatement, did a fine job.

My family, as always, gave me love.

Berkeley, California   Mark Carl Rom
April 1997

Fatal Extraction

To Cristine Rom and Alan Rocke,
wise and kind friends

CHAPTER ONE

Controversies

The Florida Dentist Case and the Centers for Disease Control and Prevention

"Open wide. This will only sting for a moment." The dentist inserts two fingers from one hand into your mouth, prying your jaws apart. Out of the corner of your eye you see the dentist reach over to the nearby stand covered with sharp tools, see the hypodermic needle raised, and then feel the eye-watering stick. Within minutes your jaw is numb, and the dentist, peering into the narrow opening into your head, can cut into the flesh and bone.

Millions of Americans have heard such words and felt that sting. On December 17, 1987, Kimberly Bergalis, a college student home for the holidays, sat in the dentist's chair as one of these millions. For her, however, the sting was more than momentary. Within two years, Bergalis was diagnosed as having AIDS. She claimed that she had contracted AIDS from her dentist, Dr. David Acer when he extracted two wisdom teeth that day in December. She died on a winter morning in 1991, when she was just twenty-three years old.

She was not alone in her tragedy. Just before Acer himself died, he published an open letter to his patients informing them that he had AIDS and had potentially exposed them to the virus. Thus far, nine other patients of the dentist have tested positive for the human immunodeficiency virus (HIV), the virus that causes AIDS. It appears that five of these people—Barbara Webb, a schoolteacher in her sixties; Richard Driskill, a married man and local contractor; Lisa Shoemaker, a traveling circus worker; John Yecs, an unemployed alcoholic; and Sherry Johnson, a high school student—also contracted HIV from Acer while receiving dental treatment.

If the claims of Bergalis and the others are right, they would be the first people known to be infected with HIV by someone providing health care. But are they? As we shall see, this case has been "one of the biggest mysteries in the annals of epidemiology" and a source of unending controversy regarding both *who* infected Bergalis and the other patients and *how* the infections happened.[1]

Getting dental care, or any medical treatment that uses sharp objects has always been an anxious experience, but if Acer indeed transmitted HIV to Bergalis and the five others, this means that patients can actually contract a grave disease while receiving medical care. Most patients—and most of us are patients from time to time— are understandably frightened by this prospect. This vision cries out for policies to protect public health in the future. As Bergalis herself concluded in a highly emotional letter published in *Newsweek* shortly before her death, "if laws are not formed to provide [patients] protection, then my suffering and death were in vain."[2]

The Bergalis story taps the special fear of AIDS that many of us feel. The issues that the case raised, however, are broader and more fundamental than those posed by this singular disease. Kimberly's death and her parents' loss would certainly not have been any less tragic if her health care provider had mortally injured her in some other way. And there are, after all, numerous ways that patients can be injured during medical care by doctors or dentists who are drunk, drugged, mentally unstable, careless, foolish, clumsy, ignorant, or otherwise incompetent. While Bergalis called for protection from AIDS, what we all really want is assurance that our health care providers will heal us and not kill us.

DID ACER DO IT? IF SO, WHAT SHOULD WE DO ABOUT IT?

In the very middle of these controversies is the Centers for Disease Control and Prevention (better known as the CDC), the federal agency that conducts medical investigations and makes public health recommendations. The CDC, for its part, has concluded that Dr. Acer did indeed infect Bergalis and at least five other patients.[3]

This conclusion has not gone unchallenged, as prominent journalists have continued to suggest that each patient contracted the disease from someone besides the dentist. Mike Wallace, on the award-winning CBS show *60 Minutes,* raised the possibility that the patients, including Bergalis, were infected through their own sexual behavior; the venerable *New York Times* and *Washington Post* carried opinion pieces that offered the same message.[4] Given the high visibility of CBS, the *Times,* and the *Post* as compared to the CDC's publication (the aptly named *Morbidity and Mortality Weekly Report,* or *MMWR*), as well as the high level of public distrust of the government, CDC officials can hardly imagine that the public agrees with them. (The CDC's investigators did take the unusual step, for the CDC, of rebutting the *60 Minutes* claims in print.[5]) As Larry Kramer, a prominent writer and AIDS activist, put it, "*60 Minutes* says one thing, the CDC another. I have more faith in *60 Minutes.* What this says is that nobody believes anything the Government is telling us about anything having to do with AIDS—how it's spread, how many people are getting it. I think that is reflected in this story's refusing to die."[6]

Some dentists agreed. The president of a Florida dental association wrote,

> After the incredible hysteria generated during the past few years after the alleged HIV contamination of six patients by Dr. David Acer, the nation deserves to receive the latest and most accurate information about this case. The CBS program *60 Minutes* provided many answers as to how these unfortunate people contracted this terrible disease. Apparently, they were victims of their own high risk behavior, not targets of an HIV-infected dentist. . . . *60 Minutes* [has] demonstrated what our profession has been saying all along: It's safe for you to go to the dentist![7]

After the CBS report aired, a column in the *New York Times* concluded that "there is now strong evidence to suspect that Dr. Acer was the innocent victim of both a witch-hunt and an inadequate investigation by the Centers for Disease Control."[8]

No less mysterious or controversial is the question of exactly how the patients became infected. The CDC investigators admit that they still do not know.[9] Some are less cautious. Mike Wallace and Stephen Barr have implied that the patients were infected through their own sexual behavior.[10] A BBC documentary concluded that Acer used contaminated dental equipment and so spread the virus to Bergalis and the others.[11] Others have argued, though with less confidence, that Acer probably infected his patients by accidentally exposing them to his blood after he injured himself while providing them dental care.[12] More spectacularly, a Barbara Walters special on the ABC show *20/20*, as well as an episode of the *Maury Povich Show*, insinuated that Acer intentionally infected—that is, murdered—his patients.[13] Former surgeon general C. Everett Koop agreed: "Unless someone comes forward with further information, we are left with no other conclusion than that Acer did it on purpose."[14]

Learning who infected the patients and how they were infected is not merely a matter of morbid curiosity. The answers are important if we are to create medical settings that are safe and secure for patients and providers alike. But just as there is little agreement about how the infections occurred, there is much conflict concerning what public policy should do about it. Most of the policy debate has nonetheless focused on the risks that HIV-positive health care workers (or, as we shall call them, HCWs) present to their patients. (Following the CDC, we define health care workers broadly as "persons, including students and trainees, whose activities involve contact with patients or with blood or other body fluids from patients in a health care setting."[15])

At first glance, the ideal policy might appear simple. Health care workers should be tested for HIV. Those who are infected should be prohibited from practicing or at least forced to disclose their infection to their patients before providing them medical care so that the patients may decide whether to accept treatment. The Bergalis family passionately favors this approach, and the public as a whole appears to agree. A 1991 Gallup poll, for example, showed that 90 percent of the public believed that all HIV-positive HCWs must disclose their condition to their patients, and 60 percent thought that HIV-infected dentists must be forbidden to practice.[16]

Many experts nonetheless consider these proposals not simple but simpleminded. They note that it is impossible to identify all infected HCWs and pointless to try. They argue that routine testing would be enormously expensive and would save few, if any, lives. (If Bergalis were murdered, the relevant fact would not be that Dr. Acer was HIV positive but that he was a psychopath.) They assert that banning HIV-positive HCWs from practice is senseless—indeed, illegal—because they have not been shown to create significant risks for their patients. Given the public's fear of HIV, we can assume that requiring these people to reveal their infection to their patients would destroy the HCWs' careers. Driving these skilled workers from practice would make health care worse, not better.

A final, most important criticism is that taking dramatic steps to lower the risk of HIV infection in medical settings misplaces our priorities. The real problem, in this view, is that patients are not endangered so much by HIV as by dangerous HCWs. Why become preoccupied with one hazardous dentist in Florida who might have gravely injured six patients by infecting them with HIV, when countless other medical providers have wounded and killed patients in other ways? An obsession with preventing HIV transmission distracts us from a more important goal: making medical care safer by reducing *all* risks.

Although doing "everything" to reduce the risks of HIV transmission in a health care setting may be unwise, doing nothing would also be unacceptable. Whatever the truth about the Florida dentist, only the most heartless policymaker could say that the government need do nothing because the risks of HIV infection from HCWs are remote. On the other hand, only the least thoughtful policymaker could say, "We will do whatever it takes" to remove HIV from the health care setting without at least pondering how much this "whatever" would cost, how effective it would be, how many lives it would save—and ruin— and whether other measures could be more effective at making medical care safer.

Did Dr. Acer infect Bergalis and the other patients, and if so, what public policies should be developed to prevent other health care workers from infecting their patients? Answering these questions would require the skills of a Sherlock and the wisdom of a Solomon; it calls for both hearts and heads. To find the answers, the American public and the medical community turned to a bureaucracy, the Centers for Disease Control and Prevention.

A BRIEF HISTORY OF THE CDC

In 1941 neither AIDS nor the Centers for Disease Control and Prevention (CDC) existed. The United States was fighting the great powers of Germany and Japan, as well as a more timeless enemy: malaria.

This was a unified national military effort, of course. The president was the commander in chief; there had been a Department of War since the nation's birth. But there was no unified national front against disease, no real "doctor in chief." The U.S. Constitution does not explicitly give either the president or Congress (or some mere agency, for that matter) the power to protect the public health; instead, it reserves this responsibility implicitly for the states.

Under the cover of World War II, a national agency was first created to lead a campaign against a single disease. The Malarial Control in War Areas agency was placed in Atlanta, Georgia, so that it would be near the southern military bases where the disease was most threatening. When the war ended, Congress was persuaded to convert this agency into a new Communicable Disease Center so that it could continue its work on malaria and other diseases. With a token payment of $10, the government bought fifteen acres of land on Clifton Road, outside Atlanta, for the CDC's new headquarters. Malaria had brought the agency to the South, and it is there still.[17]

Over the years the CDC and its mission expanded as it became the federal agency responsible for monitoring health issues and providing "pragmatic guidance" for local action.[18] The nickname "CDC" is a symbol both of its new responsibilities and its enduring commitment to controlling diseases. Over time, its full name has evolved from the Communicable Disease Center to the Center for Disease Control (1970) to the Centers (plural) for Disease Control (1980) to the Centers for Disease Control and Prevention (1992). Throughout, its acronym has remained the same. Its monitoring responsibilities have involved detective work known, in the health community, as surveillance and epidemiological research. To train its medical detectives, the CDC in 1951 established its Epidemic Intelligence Service. Its graduates, the CDC's surveillance officers, have become the agency's rapid-response team for health emergencies, at home and abroad.

In the year of our nation's bicentennial, for example, a mysterious illness struck down 182 people attending an American Legion conference, killing 29. The CDC's surveillance officers were sent in to find the cause. After 73,000 hours of work over several intensive months, the CDC solved the puzzle: the deaths were caused by a bacteria the CDC named *Legionella pneumophilia,* or "Legionnaires' disease."[19]

Once the CDC learns the cause of an epidemic, the agency then attempts to control it by offering "pragmatic guidance," which, normally, is just that. The CDC has no legal power to compel anybody to do anything: it is neither a regulatory nor a law enforcement agency. Like a doctor, it can only advise. And like a doctor, its advice only does good if the patient—such as hospitals or local health agencies—wants to follow it and is actually able to do so. In the early years, the CDC's guidance was typically followed, and the agency developed a quiet reputation for expertise.

Most often, the CDC investigated outbreaks of communicable diseases, determined the causes of these outbreaks, developed recommendations for preventing them, and issued these public health guidelines with little controversy in its publication, the *MMWR*. In this way the CDC took on polio in 1955, influenza in 1957, and smallpox in 1966. The CDC even participated in the quarantine of Neil Armstrong and his crew as they returned from the first moon landing in 1969.

It seemed that the CDC's reputation would continue to grow with its successes. By the late 1970s the CDC was able to announce the last case of smallpox in the world and the last case of wild polio virus in the United States. A new vaccine for the hepatitis B virus had been developed at the end of the decade, promising to save millions of lives, and the CDC had been instrumental in conducting the definitive study of the virus's epidemiology. Perhaps some people even dared to hope, as the 1980s began, that the end of the deadly infectious diseases was at hand.

But then, in early 1981, puzzling cases of rare ailments started appearing in New York and California. In Los Angeles alone, five homosexual men had developed *Pneumocystis pneumonia,* a most unusual and life-threatening condition. Two physicians—one a CDC surveillance officer—wrote a worried summary about the potential link between these ailments and some aspect of the homosexual lifestyle or sexual transmission and submitted it to the agency for immediate publication in the *MMWR*.

Dr. James Curran, the chief of research in the CDC's Sexually Transmitted Diseases (STD) Division, reviewed the manuscript. Curran had spent his entire career in the CDC, joining it in 1970 when at age twenty-six he finished medical school, and he was no stranger to strange venereal diseases, yet his penciled comments on the manuscript revealed both medical excitement and alarm: "Hot Stuff. Hot Stuff."[20] Within two weeks the *MMWR* would carry the innocuously entitled report "*Pneumocystis Pneumonia*—Los Angeles," the first published report of the disease soon to be known as AIDS.[21]

Shortly before the article was published, Curran and Dr. Harold Jaffe (another CDC veteran) attended a sexually transmitted disease conference in San Diego. They announced the forthcoming *MMWR* report and asked whether others at the conference knew of similar cases. Some had. Returning to Atlanta, Curran and Jaffe (together with Dr. Mary Guinan) suggested to their bosses that this problem needed more study; they were given permission to drop most of their normal duties and set up a task force to do so. They quickly learned of additional cases (who often also had Kaposi's sarcoma, a previously rare form of cancer) and published a second report on the new ailment.[22]

Curran, Jaffe, Guinan, and a small group of other investigators moved to collect additional information on this extraordinary disease, first by calling doctors and health departments and then by going to Los Angeles, San Francisco, and New York City for personal interviews with those afflicted. These lengthy interviews helped the task force begin to piece together the common elements linking the cases. The results were alarming. Curran and Jaffe reported back to their boss: "This is a huge problem and we have to get going on it."[23] The entire STD division stopped its existing research and focused solely on the mysterious plague.

In the coming years Curran, Jaffe, and others within the CDC scraped for resources, and there were never enough, to help them understand and control the surging epidemic. Each day the news grew worse. It first became clear that the disease was becoming widespread among homosexual men, suggesting that it was an infectious disease. Then it started showing up among IV drug users, further evidence that it was a bloodborne illness. The task force knew what this meant: if the disease was spread through blood, those who received blood transfusions were at risk.

In the summer of 1982, first one, then two, then a third hemophiliac—neither homosexuals nor IV drug users—developed the by now familiar symptoms. The CDC announced the news in its typically mild manner: "Although the course of the severe immune dysfunction is unknown, the occurrence among the three hemophiliac cases suggests the possible transmission of an agent through blood products."[24] While publicly merely "suggesting" that it was "possible" that transfusions could transmit AIDS, the task force members were convinced that transfusions actually did and that the problem would become huge if it were not checked. Yet Curran was unable to persuade a special meeting of blood banks, the Hemophilia Foundation, the National Gay

Task Force, or the Food and Drug Administration (which regulated the blood banks) that there was a serious problem; they rejected his evidence as insufficient.[25]

Then a baby in San Francisco developed symptoms of AIDS after receiving blood transfusions from a man who had died from the disease. And four more hemophiliacs developed symptoms. And four young children, born to mothers who were IV drug users, became seriously ill. According to Jaffe, "all these things that represented our worst nightmares were actually happening."[26]

The CDC thus convened another meeting soon after the first to convince blood bankers and others that urgent actions were needed to improve the safety of the blood supply. Once again, the CDC was rebuffed. As Jaffe put it, "much to our surprise, people did not believe these cases and were not convinced. . . . There was this tremendous denial of the problem. We were stunned. It seemed so clear."[27] But another CDC official provided an alternate perspective:

> [The] CDC was going alone. We had a terrible time convincing other people [about] things that had to be done quickly. You can't blame people [for resisting]. CDC was calling the shots on almost no evidence—educated guesses rather than proof. We did not have proof that [AIDS] was bloodborne; we had five hemophiliacs and two or three blood transfusion cases. We did not have proof it was a contagious agent; we had epidemiological evidence suggesting it.[28]

Indeed, just a week before this meeting to warn of the hazards in the blood supply, Jaffe had gone on record trying to calm the public: "The risk to the general population [from blood transfusions] is quite small and the need to receive blood far outweighs the concerns about AIDS."[29] By the time that the blood banks began making serious efforts to clean up the blood supply, over 150 recipients of blood transfusions had developed AIDS and thousands more had been infected. To Curran and Jaffe, who knew the dangers as well as anyone, this must have been a frustrating time.

The CDC's warning to the blood banks foreshadowed the case of the Florida dentist. Once again, Curran, Jaffe, and the CDC had limited evidence, weak powers, and a public health problem of enormous significance. Yet there was a critically important difference between the two episodes. The CDC officials believed that, unless the blood banks acted swiftly to control HIV, thousands of patients were likely to become infected through tainted transfusions. In contrast, the CDC officials expected that few patients were likely to be infected by their HCWs, and so dramatic changes in health policies were unwarranted. In both episodes they had to impress those providing health care with the need to recognize and act on an important medical problem, while at the same time they had to keep the public from panicking. Yet in the case of the blood banks, the greatest risks were to public health; in the case of the Florida dentist, the greatest risk was to public confidence in the health system.

WHAT ROLE DID THE CDC PLAY?

It was the CDC's responsibility to find out *who* infected the patients, to determine *how* they were infected, and to decide *what* our nation should do about it. We will shadow the CDC to discover what they knew—and to see whether others knew more. By doing so, we can learn *what* the CDC did to accomplish its goals, *why* it did these things, and *how* it might have done them better.

The story of the fatal extraction has been a mystery without a proper ending. Acquaintances invariably tell me that they've heard about this case and then confide that "the dentist murdered his patients, didn't he?," or "I heard that he used contaminated tools," or "the patients caught HIV through risky sex, right?" This range of responses is perhaps inevitable, since this case caught the attention of the American public as few other medical stories have.

Yet the story fragments that are remembered are the sensational ones. The media are inclined to reject the CDC's official account that Acer infected at least six of his patients but that the precise manner of infection is unknown. Murder, tainted tools, and sexual activity have all been variously reported to national audiences as responsible for the infections. These reports, moreover, have focused almost exclusively on the beginning of the story (did Acer infect the patients and, if so, how?) rather than on the ending (what should we do about it?) or on the big picture (how can we make the health care setting safer and more secure for patients and medical professionals alike?).

That the media missed almost entirely the story of what the CDC did to answer these questions should not be surprising. Murder, scandal, and sex are telegenic in ways that bureaucratic behavior is not. The CDC did little to change this balance; they have been reluctant to grant interviews on this case and reticent in offering their personal views.

The CDC's health officials have presented their side of the story in official announcements (such as the *MMWR*) and in journal articles. These publications—especially those subject to review by outside experts—have been informative and solid.[30] Still, they suffer two flaws inherent in government publications. First, they virtually always conceal as much as they reveal; indeed, the CDC provided only brief summaries of its investigations in the *MMWR*. More important, those who distrust the government are unlikely to be persuaded by official publications. Governmental agencies find themselves in the unenviable position of being doubted simply because they are part of the government.

A more difficult task than determining whether the CDC arrived at the correct conclusion is to clarify why the CDC officials did what they did. "Bureaucratic politics" is the explanation I propose. This may seem like an unfortunate phrase that describes precisely what is wrong with the CDC: bureaucracy and politics. But my meaning is not pejorative; I use the term to describe why individuals behave as they do in their roles as governmental officials.

This behavior is influenced by the agency itself: how the CDC is organized, what its main tasks are, what kind of culture it has, and how it defines its mission.[31] Bureaucratic politics are also affected by the relationships that the CDC maintained with the public, other agencies, and the broader political environment. Ultimately, however, all bureaucratic politics involve the actions of individuals, affected as they are by their own training, experiences, beliefs, and motivations.[32]

The latter merits special attention. The conventional wisdom (as expressed by journalists and scholars) is that those involved in politics—bureaucrats, politicians, citizens—are motivated almost entirely by their own self-interest. But this is more conventional than wise. Saint Teresas are rare, of course; few people involved in politics, or anything else for that matter, are purely self-sacrificial. Yet it is needlessly cynical to believe that people are always out just to get their own. Perhaps those active in politics—including those involved in the case of the Florida dentist—are seeking to produce a society that is better for all and not just for themselves. The fact that they often disagree can simply mean that they have different visions of what this society should be. Just as we probably believe that what we seek in our political activities is best for the country, those who disagree with us might also believe that their way will best serve the public's interests.[33]

The final, toughest task is to consider how the CDC might have done its jobs better. That it needed to do so might seem self-evident. No one has praised the CDC's handling of the Bergalis case; rather, the criticism comes from all sides. The CDC has been blamed both for doubting too long Bergalis's allegations that she contracted HIV from Acer and for going public too quickly with its report that Acer probably did infect her. The CDC has been criticized both for creating hysteria about the possibility that health care workers could infect patients with HIV and for misleading the public about the true risks of such transmissions. The CDC has been chastised both for precipitously issuing too harsh recommendations to minimize the possibilities of patients contracting HIV from HCWs and for issuing unduly mild guidelines only after long delay.

If some believe that the CDC acted responsibly and wisely in its efforts to develop public health recommendations for HIV and HCWs, they do so quietly. Instead, the CDC officials are almost universally referred to by partisans in this case in the harshest personal way—as being corrupt or cowardly, if not wicked. Sanford Kuvin, Bergalis's medical advisor, who advocates mandatory testing of HCWs for HIV and practice restrictions for those who are infected, argues that "the CDC does not have the testicular fortitude [to adopt these policies]. . . . They have become corrupted by politics."[34] Others who opposed such policies voiced similar concerns about the CDC to me (although not for the record). Even some within the CDC share the opinion that the agency has become too politicized. Don Francis, a CDC official involved early in its AIDS work, claimed in his retirement speech that the "CDC lost sight of its role as an advocate for the public's health and inadvertently became a servant of politicians who were uninhibited by knowledge, experience, or wisdom."[35] Harsher still, but hardly unique, are the words of one observer quoted in the *Congressional Record*:

> She is dying because the political and public-health systems are more interested in protecting the wayward, the deviant, and the promiscuous than the upright. . . . She was like a lamb led to the slaughter. The whole political, medical and public-health system . . . joined in a conspiracy of silence to shield Dr. Acer's deadly disease and allow hundreds of patients to be exposed to his infection. If this is not cold-blooded, deliberate dereliction of duty on a massive scale, I don't know what is.[36]

But in fact, as we shall see, health officials struggled to create policies that would genuinely improve public health; the inability to devise a perfect solution reveals the difficulty of the duty more than the motivations of the participants. The kind of inflammatory language often used in American politics unfortunately made these struggles harder than they needed to be.

That the CDC has angered virtually everyone concerned about HIV in the health care workplace does not necessarily mean that it did the wrong things. It is possible that no set of policies would have been widely popular, especially as the issues involved the highly contentious disputes of highly passionate advocates. Perhaps compromises that leave all advocates displeased are the best that can be hoped for, particularly when no advocates will be pleased unless their view triumphs. But it might at least have been possible for the CDC to develop its policies in such a way that partisans on all sides commended its efforts if not its results. To do so, the CDC needed the clearest possible understanding of what actually happened in Dr. David Acer's dental clinic. Let us now follow the agency officials there.

CHAPTER TWO

Sex
The Government Investigates the Dentist's Patients

───〰〰〰───

Nikki knows sex and drugs. It was her job. As the surveillance manager for the Palm Beach County Health Unit, District Nine, in Florida's Department of Health and Rehabilitative Services (HRS) at the time that Kimberly Bergalis was diagnosed with AIDS, Nikki Economou investigated individuals to determine how they had contracted AIDS. She left me little doubt that she knew how to do this.

Economou, like her counterparts in state health departments around the country, had numerous responsibilities for slowing the spread of AIDS. One job was to contact the sexual partners of persons with AIDS so that they could be tested for HIV, receive counseling about health care, and be informed about what they needed to do to keep from spreading the disease (or contracting it, if their blood tests indicated they were not infected). Another duty was to learn how persons with "no identified risks" of contracting AIDS became infected. She did these things because Florida, like the other states, had decided that AIDS posed a risk to the public health.

AIDS REPORTING AND RISK FACTORS

Bureaucrats do not know and really do not care about every time you sneeze. Only certain diseases are "reportable," meaning that when a physician learns that a person has this disease the physician must give this information to public health officials. But it is not the federal government that determines which diseases are reportable, even though the "public health" may seem to be a national concern. One national association, the Conference of State and Territorial Epidemiologists (CSTE), does make recommendations about which diseases should be reportable in every state, but it has no statutory power to enforce its recommendations. (The CSTE is a membership organization comprising the leading epidemiologists in every state.) Only the states have the legal authority to make diseases reportable and to decide what information about these diseases must be reported to state officials. As anyone who has traveled the country could guess, the states vary widely regarding which diseases are reported, which officials must be notified, what information must be collected, and how vigorously these reports are collected.

The CDC does monitor reportable diseases around the country for the federal government. Although the CDC tells the states what information it would like to receive about their reportable diseases, it has no authority to compel the states to submit this information or to punish them if they do not. The CDC consequently accepts information in a wide variety of forms, as some states have the individual physicians or hospitals submit reports while other states have more centralized reporting systems. Although the CDC has developed standard reporting forms for HIV and AIDS and encourages the states to use them, it does not necessarily receive standardized information at specific intervals from the states.

When Bergalis was diagnosed, AIDS was a reportable disease in Florida and all the other states (HIV, in contrast, was a reportable disease in less than half of them).[1] When a person is diagnosed with AIDS in Florida, the attending physician must report basic information to the state health department. The department compiles this information and periodically sends it—minus the patient's name and address—to the CDC in Atlanta. These reports include various clinical and laboratory data and, of special interest here, information about the patient's "risk factors."

HIV is a bloodborne disease. For a person to contract HIV and thus develop AIDS, that person must be directly exposed to the blood, semen, or vaginal fluids of a person with HIV. (These are often euphemistically labeled "bodily fluids." Sweat, spit, and tears also fall into this category and even can contain trace amounts of HIV, but they do not create real risks of infection.) The most common ways in which such exposures occur are through unprotected sexual contact—particularly those likely to expose semen to blood—and through sharing the needles used to inject illicit drugs. As a result, if an HIV-positive person has had sexual contact with a homosexual or bisexual male, injected illicit drugs, received blood transfusions, or had sexual contact with any individual who has done these things, that person is said to have "identified risk" factors. If the HIV-positive person denies such exposures, that person is reported as having "no identified risk" (NIR) factors.

The key information needed to trace the spread of AIDS concerns the patient's potential exposures to HIV—that is, the ways in which a person came into contact with infected blood, semen, or vaginal fluid. To learn about these risk factors, the attending physician asks each patient diagnosed with AIDS how they believe they contracted the disease. This information is placed in the AIDS case report. The CDC counts the most common methods of HIV transmission on the basis of these reports. These methods differ for men and women. Around the time that Bergalis was diagnosed, the risk factors identified most often for males were

· Homosexual or bisexual contact (65 percent of the cases)

· Intravenous (IV) drug use (19 percent)

· Homosexual or bisexual contact and IV drug use (7 percent)

· Receipt of blood transfusions, blood components, or tissue (3 percent)

· Other or undetermined modes (3 percent)

· Heterosexual contact (2 percent)

For females the most frequently cited risk factors were

· IV drug use (51 percent)

· Heterosexual contact (33 percent)

· Receipt of blood transfusions, blood components, or tissue (8 percent)

· Other or undetermined (7 percent)[2]

These rankings did not necessarily indicate the true frequency of the various modes of transmission because unfortunately many persons with HIV had more than one risk factor. With the exception of males who have had sexual contact with other males and used IV drugs, however, only one risk factor is identified for each person diagnosed. (The CDC now reports annually the percentage of cases with multiple risk factors.) This is because the CDC believes that the risk factors fall into a hierarchy. For example, if a male admitted to having sex with another man or if a female acknowledged IV drug use, then heterosexual contact by either of these persons would not typically be identified as a risk factor. Once a single risk factor had been identified, that person was assumed to have contracted HIV in that way. As a result, the factors at the bottom of the hierarchy tended to be under-reported and the factors at the top overreported. Remember, too, that while these reports revealed the risky behaviors of persons testing positive, the reports did not *demonstrate* that these persons were in fact infected through these behaviors. It is possible, after all, for a man to engage in homosexual activity, inject drugs—and still be infected through a blood transfusion.

That there is an "other or undetermined" category does not necessarily imply that there are additional risk factors that are yet to be discovered. "Other" refers to the few persons who have developed AIDS after exposure to HIV-infected blood within the health care setting or in some other bizarre way. (At the time Bergalis was diagnosed, for example, about forty HCWs had been infected with HIV through accidental exposure in the workplace. Since then, one man contracted the virus when a prostitute bit him severely.) "Undetermined" cases are those whose mode of exposure to HIV has not yet been identified. This group includes persons who were still under investigation; those who have died, were lost to follow-up, or refused to be interviewed; and individuals whose mode of exposure to HIV remained undetermined even after investigation.[3]

Most "no identified risk" (NIR) cases eventually are reclassified when one or more of the risk factors are found.[4] Some cases are classified as NIR simply because the infected person was not given the interview about risk factors. Other persons with AIDS initially deny that they have had behavioral risk factors but, when reinterviewed, admit to having put themselves at risk. More rarely, a patient will continue to deny having risk factors for AIDS, yet evidence is found to contradict these denials. Still, the numbers are daunting. Through July 1991, for instance, there were 12,329 AIDS cases in the United States that were initially reported as having undetermined risk factors. Even after follow-up information was collected, 491 individuals were still specified as "no risk identified or other" source of infection. Again, this does not imply that HIV is spread in unknown ways; it does suggest that health officials find it difficult to find the cause of infection for each and every case.

The difficulty of identifying and corroborating the risk factors for females is of special importance in the Acer case, involving, as it did, four female patients. As the list of risk factors indicates, the vast majority (95 percent) of male exposures can be traced to conduct (such as having sex with another man, using IV drugs, or receiving blood transfusions) about which the infected male himself has firsthand knowledge. In other words, the surveillance office could determine the risk factors of males by asking them, "Did *you* have any of these risk factors?" In contrast, a substantial proportion (33 percent) of AIDS cases for females could be traced to the conduct of *their* heterosexual contacts; the female may only have secondhand information about the risky behaviors of these men or even be entirely unaware of them. For many females, the officer would need to ask, "Did *your partner* have any of these risk factors?" In the absence of corroboration, this secondhand information is much less solid than that obtained firsthand.

If an individual declares certain behaviors, no further efforts to identify risk factors are usually considered necessary. If an HIV-positive male acknowledges having homosexual or bisexual contact, for example, or an HIV-positive female admits IV drug use, or if either a male or a female concedes having sexual contact with homosexuals, bisexuals, or IV drug users, this is typically considered sufficient evidence of how the person contracted the virus. As far as the surveillance office is concerned, such admissions close the case.

Heterosexual contact, in contrast, is not considered to be adequate indication of how transmission occurred. Heterosexual contact is considered a risky behavior only if the person's heterosexual contacts are themselves known to be bisexuals, IV drug users, or HIV-positive. A surveillance officer would thus consider an HIV-positive male having multiple heterosexual contacts with unknown individuals as having no identified risk factors, but an otherwise identical individual who acknowledged even one homosexual contact would be considered to have an identified risk factor.

TRACING THE SPREAD OF HIV

Determining the risk factors of persons with HIV can pose tremendous challenges to the surveillance officer. Individuals may be reluctant to describe highly personal, stigmatized, or illegal activities (such as sexual behavior or drug use) to a government official. They are certainly not compelled to do so and may have a variety of motives for concealing or denying the truth.

Information about sexual behavior or drug use is also typically difficult to corroborate. The reasons are partially physical: material evidence of such activities is often fleeting, witnesses rare, and memories bad. Semen washes off and leaves no footprints. Junkies do not shoot up with the authorities. The lustful do not invite the (official) photographers to document their behavior. And not everyone learns and remembers the name of that sexual encounter, especially if the night of passion began with an evening of drinking.

Highly personal information can also be difficult to confirm because state and federal laws protect individual privacy.[5] Suppose that HIV-positive Person X claimed to have had sex with Person Y. A surveillance office might naturally want to corroborate this by asking Person Y, "Did you have sex with Person X?" This question, posed this way, virtually invites Person Y to retaliate against X for spreading this personal information. Such direct questioning is thus an illegal invasion of privacy in Florida and other states.

Surveillance officers, facing such confidentiality laws, conduct contact tracing with what is called "cluster interviewing." In cluster interviews, the officer would ask Person Y something like "With whom have you had sex?," hoping that Person X would be mentioned. If Person Y does not acknowledge having had sexual contact with Person X, it's tough luck for the officer, unless other substantiation can be obtained. Cluster interviewing would not be too difficult if everyone cooperated with the officer, knew the facts, remembered them, and told the truth about them. Everyone doesn't.

The case of a real "Person X" from the Washington, D.C., metropolitan area illustrates some of the difficulties AIDS surveillance officers face.[6] The case began when Person X ("Tiffany"), a fifteen-year-old pregnant woman, tested HIV positive. When interviewed by her physician, she denied using IV drugs or receiving blood transfusions. She did report having sex with six male teenagers, four of whom lived in her apartment complex, during the previous two years. Her partners, she revealed, rarely wore condoms. Tiffany's physician called the Prince Georges (Maryland) County Health Department to report the diagnosis and this information to its surveillance officers.

Good investigators begin with their strongest leads. Although it was possible that Tiffany had been infected through IV drug use or blood transfusions and not through sexual contact, she had admitted having sex and denied shooting drugs. Jan Scott, the principal investigator in this case, thus focused her inquiry on the six young men Tiffany had named, and contacted them all. Four of them came in for blood tests that showed that they had not been infected. One youth ignored repeated requests to be tested.

The sixth youth ("Steven") tested HIV positive. As Scott remembered it, this sixteen-year-old learned he was infected with HIV "with wide eyes that seemed to stare at nothing in particular. . . . He seemed really scared and small. He didn't say much. He didn't ask questions. He listened to what I had to say and then he asked if he could be excused."[7]

But after giving Steven the news that he had contracted an apparently incurable disease, Scott still had to ask this youth about the most intimate details of his personal life. Steven said that he had not used IV drugs or received blood transfusions, and he guessed that he had had about five sexual partners. He did not name Tiffany as one of these partners, however. As Steven did not report Tiffany as a sexual contact, Scott was left wondering how many other contacts Steven failed to report. Steven could not remember the name of one of these contacts (although the description he gave did not match that of Tiffany), and Scott was not able to locate another one of the women. A third contact tested negative, and a fourth person refused to meet with Scott.

The fifth woman ("Keisha"), another sixteen-year-old, was located. She also tested positive for HIV. Keisha, in turn, denied shooting drugs or receiving transfusions and stated that she had had sex with three individuals, including Steven. Neither of the two remaining partners could be located and tested. One of them was murdered before Scott could contact him. The other one lived in a different jurisdiction in which Scott had no authority to work; the information about this case was passed to a surveillance officer in that jurisdiction, who was not able to locate him. Having exhausted all leads, this investigation came to an end.

Scott ultimately attempted to trace all the sexual partners of three individuals who proved to be HIV positive. She heard about eleven partners, although an undetermined number of others existed. We can be certain that at least one person (Steven) did not mention all his sexual contacts, and we have no way of knowing whether the other individuals actually listed all their partners. Six of the eleven were not tested either because the infected individuals could not remember these people's names, they could not be located, they lived in a different jurisdiction, they refused to cooperate, or they were dead.

Scott knew when she reached a dead end that all potential routes of infection had not been traced. It is impossible that Tiffany, Steven, and Keisha only infected each other; there must have been some unidentified person who introduced HIV into this group. Still, she might have drawn some tentative conclusions. As the data indicate that men are more likely to infect women through sex than vice versa, and because both Tiffany and Keisha reported having sex with Steven, and because Steven was the only one of the traceable contacts for either patient who was HIV positive, it looks like Steven transmitted HIV to Tiffany and Keisha, while he in turn was infected by some other person.

Yet several puzzles remain. If Steven was *not* the source of HIV, did Tiffany or Keisha lie when they denied that they used IV drugs? Did they have other sexual partners whom they forgot or chose not to reveal? If, on the other hand, Steven was the source of the virus for Tiffany and Keisha, then how did *he* contract it? Did Steven not reveal that he had a sexual experience with one or more males—a likely prospect, as it is not uncommon for men to have sex with other men and deny it—or that he was an IV drug user?[8] Or had one untraced contact served as the ultimate source of the virus for this group?

Despite the unanswered questions from this case, it was still a relatively uncontroversial investigation. All the infected persons admitted behaviors that potentially put them at risk for contracting HIV, and the surveillance officers had the full names of at least some of the sexual partners. But what happens when a person with HIV makes no such admissions?

THE KIMBERLY BERGALIS INVESTIGATION

On December 4, 1989, Kimberly Bergalis checked into the Indian River Hospital in her home, Fort Pierce, Florida, with a severe case of pneumonia. She was diagnosed as having AIDS. Two days later, on Wednesday, during a standard medical interview for persons with AIDS, Bergalis denied using IV drugs, receiving blood transfusions, and having sexual partners. Bergalis did note, however, that she had received treatment from a dentist whom she believed had AIDS. Because she denied having engaged in any behaviors that would have put her in danger of contracting AIDS, she was listed as a "no identified risk" case when her physician submitted this report to the health department in West Palm Beach. The following Thursday, December 14, Economou visited Bergalis at the hospital for the first of what would be many interviews.[9]

Economou was an experienced surveillance officer. Trained as an epidemiologist by the CDC, she had been working for the Florida Department of Health and Rehabilitative Services for eighteen years, before becoming responsible for AIDS surveillance in the fifteen counties comprising District Nine. Prior to her District Nine posting, Economou had worked at the Immunodeficiency Clinic at the University of South Florida for four years.[10] A central responsibility of her job as surveillance officer was to identify the risk factors of NIR cases.

Over the course of six hours, Economou interviewed Bergalis, gradually administering an eighteen-page questionnaire developed by the CDC for AIDS cases. The questionnaire contained queries concerning Bergalis's family background, health history, and sexual activities or drug use. In this lengthy interview—conducted one-on-one—Bergalis reiterated that she had done nothing to contract HIV. Within the first hour, however, Bergalis implicated her dentist as a possible source of infection.[11] At the conclusion of this interview, Economou wrote:

Patient was alert, intelligent, and cooperative. We discussed all issues of sexuality and drugs—she detailed her "physical relationships" with people she dated while in school. Moderate petting is as close as I could come to describing her activities. No mutual masturbation; no sexual contact and never any drugs. She drinks a wine cooler every couple of weeks. I recommended that all family members get tested (to rule out any possibilities). They agreed. Thorough physical by her physician shows her hymen to be intact and no signs of rectal or oral sexual interaction. She has agreed to being reinterviewed by me again.[12]

(The CDC and the HRS have not released their case notes or any other confidential information from their inquiry to the public. Any files that contain such information and are cited in this book were obtained from the law offices of Montgomery and Larmoyeux, legal counsel to the Bergalis family.)

Immediately afterward, Economou also conducted a private interview with Bergalis's mother, Anna. The next day, Economou called the state HRS office in Tallahassee to tell them that she had a "hot case." This was the first time that Economou had called the state headquarters about an NIR case.

What was Economou to make of Bergalis's claims? Some statements were credible on the surface. It would be relatively easy to confirm that Bergalis had not received any blood transfusions. It was also difficult for Economou to believe that Bergalis injected drugs. While appearances can deceive, few persons fitting Bergalis's demographic description (female, middle class, southern, college student) were junkies, and she certainly didn't seem to be one to Economou.

Regarding Bergalis's sexual behavior, on the other hand, Economou had reasons to be skeptical. While Bergalis denied having had sexual contacts, the vast majority (about 80 percent) of women who attend college have had sexual intercourse by the time they are as old as Bergalis was, with each woman having had on average three sexual partners.[13] Moreover, even "virgins"—those who have not engaged in vaginal intercourse—can be at some risk of contracting HIV through sexual behavior. (For example, one study of the sexual practices of almost one thousand virgins between the ninth and twelfth grades found that about 10 percent had engaged in fellatio without a condom, a sexual activity creating a small risk of transmitting HIV.[14]) Economou also learned that Bergalis's family was devoutly Catholic—a religion that views premarital sex as a sin of some importance. Economou furthermore knew that most NIR cases are eventually reclassified when a risk factor is later identified, typically when the person ultimately acknowledges having some risky sexual behavior. Given these statistics and these beliefs, even a skilled questioner like Economou was likely to surmise that unless Bergalis's statements could be verified, this NIR case had undisclosed sexual partners.

Yet Economou was in a precarious position. In order to obtain accurate and complete information about Bergalis's sexual behavior, Economou needed Bergalis to trust her. This trust might have to be violated, however. Economou would not be able to keep any sexual secrets Bergalis might tell her but would need to report them as part of the case file, and thus her parents would inevitably learn of or deduce them. Bergalis recognized this dilemma. As her father stated,

> Kim saw through [Economou] right away. Nikki became a "friend" only to learn any intimate details that she theorized Kim had not told her on that first interview. She wasn't Kim's friend. She was working for the CDC [actually, the HRS], and she was using "friendship" as a way to find out why Kim had lied—only Kim hadn't lied. She told them the truth.[15]

As it turned out, however, Bergalis did not tell the entire truth during the first interview; she had had sexual activity beyond what she acknowledged then. She should not be blamed for her reticence; it would be truly amazing if any American would tell some government official all the details of his or her personal life on first acquaintance. But this does suggest that however truthful Bergalis was, Economou had the duty to continue meeting with her until the details could be verified.

The Bergalis case was not Economou's only responsibility, of course, but was one of many cases that she was tracking. Economou consequently began scanning for evidence while she went about the other parts of her job. As she did when investigating any case, she kept her eyes open for potential links, wondering whether some other HIV-positive person would acknowledge having sex with Bergalis. Economou screened state computers to see if Bergalis had been reported as having some other sexually transmitted disease; in Florida, syphilis and several other sexually transmitted diseases are, like AIDS, reportable. Nothing turned up.

All the while, Bergalis's NIR case file was slowly working its way toward the CDC's attention. There were, as one would expect, formal procedures for its progress. Palm Beach County routinely sent its AIDS surveillance reports, including the NIR cases, to the administrative offices of the Florida Department of Health and Rehabilitative Services (HRS) in Tallahassee. The state office, in turn, would collect and collate all its district surveillance reports and forward them to the CDC headquarters in Atlanta. The CDC receives AIDS reports from every state, compiles them, and then publishes them monthly in its *HIV/AIDS Surveillance Report*. But paper sometimes flows slowly. As the CDC has admitted, "reporting delays vary widely by geographic area and have been several years in some cases."[16] In 1989, the typical reporting delay (the time between when the patient was diagnosed with AIDS and when the CDC records the case report) was three months.

The sluggish paper flow into the CDC headquarters may have been just about the only typical part of this case. Bergalis was diagnosed with AIDS on December 4 and was interviewed by Economou on December 14. About ten days after this interview, Economou sent her case report (as well as others from the district) to the state office, which stamped it "Received" on December 28, 1989. It is not clear when this file was sent to Atlanta, but it seems that it sat in Tallahassee for at least a couple of weeks. In Atlanta, it then sat around for a few more. (The CDC had a vacancy in its surveillance office at that time, so the NIR reports stacked up until that position was filled in February.) Finally, the Bergalis case was entered into the CDC's files as one of the more than one hundred NIR cases reported each month.

But the Bergalis case actually came to the CDC's attention in a much more human way. The CDC hosts periodic conferences for AIDS surveillance officers so that they could learn more about the spread of AIDS, hear about new techniques to control the epidemic, and, of course, swap stories about life and death in the field. At that year's conference (held on February 28, 1990, in Atlanta) an informal conversation developed among Economou, Spencer Lieb (an epidemiologist with the HRS in Tallahassee), and a CDC official. Economou described the puzzling circumstances of the Bergalis case and admitted "I'm running out of angles."[17] At some point in the following weeks, the Florida HRS formally invited the CDC to join the investigation of the Bergalis case. On Monday, March 27, 1990, Carol Ciesielski, in charge of NIR investigations for the CDC, flew to Florida to join Economou in her increasingly mysterious research.

The CDC is called into a state to conduct a field investigation perhaps 150 times each year. Usually a hospital, with the approval of the state health department, invites the CDC to investigate an outbreak of some infectious disease. In response, the CDC will dispatch an "Epi-Aids" (epidemiological assistance) officer (or team) to the hospital to determine how the outbreak occurred. Because these requests happen so often, the CDC has a well-developed way for handling them—indeed, at the time of the Bergalis case, it had a sixty-seven-page guidebook.[18] This Epi-Aids manual provided guidance for conducting and reporting these investigations, from the initial request ("Outline and Checklist for Originating Epi-Aids Missions"), through the various reporting requirements (how to file Epi–1, 2, and 3 reports), to the handling of freedom of information requests for the results. The CDC's trained Epidemic Intelligence Service (EIS) officers are to conduct these investigations.

Ciesielski had been an Epidemic Intelligence Service officer for the CDC during 1985–1987, before she started working on AIDS surveillance for the agency. At the time of the Bergalis case, she was in charge of the NIR inquiries and was also developing a system to detect and report cases in which HCWs had contracted HIV occupationally. As a result, she was deeply involved in the issues surrounding HIV transmission in medical settings. There was no question that she would be the one to travel to Florida.

Ciesielski first interviewed Bergalis on March 28 while walking on Bergalis's favorite beach near her home. Ciesielski did not administer a formal questionnaire but instead engaged Bergalis in a wide-ranging conversation to identify possible exposures to HIV. In this interview, Ciesielski learned a few new items of potential importance. Bergalis had become "blood sisters" with a friend in ninth grade (1983) by pricking each other's finger and using a drop of blood to seal an envelope containing a pledge of lifelong support. (The CDC found the childhood friend and checked on her health; she was fine.) Ciesielski also noted that Bergalis "shared razors with dormmates on occasion in college. No one known HIV positive. Patient recalls going dancing with friends, cut foot on broken glass on dance floor. Cleaned it up in the restroom."[19] Neither of these leads led to anything. None of Bergalis's college friends, moreover, were known to be HIV positive. At the end of the interview, Ciesielski obtained a sample of Bergalis's blood. Although Ciesielski was a medical doctor and quite qualified to draw blood samples, Kimberly's mother (a nurse) actually drew them.

The following day, Ciesielski and Economou interviewed dentist David Acer at his home in Stuart. By this time, Acer was suffering from full-blown AIDS (he would die in August). He had retired from dentistry the previous year, in July 1989, as his health deteriorated. Ciesielski informed him that a patient (she of course did not mention Bergalis by name) had mentioned him as a possible source of HIV infection. Economou thought that Acer looked "blown away" by this news, asking, "How could you take someone's word for it?" But he cooperated fully with his interviewers. (Ironically, while Bergalis complained that the investigators did not trust her enough, Acer perceived that they believed her too much.) Acer briefly described his dental practice, claiming that he used proper infection control practices and wore latex gloves while treating patients. He did not remember ever severely cutting himself while giving treatment, although he conceded that he sometimes stuck himself while recapping the needles used to administer anesthetic. He expressed great concern for the infected patient. He agreed to share his patient records with the health authorities, while noting that most of them had been dispersed after he sold his practice; he had kept only the records of the patients who had not paid their bills. Most important, he allowed Ciesielski to withdraw three small vials of blood for genetic testing. After about an hour, the interview ended.

This, unfortunately, was to be Acer's only interview. The next day, he called Economou to tell her that on the advice of his family, he would be represented by a lawyer in all future contacts with health officials.

This interview, which must have seemed uneventful at the time, has turned into one of the most important but also most heavily criticized parts of the CDC's investigation. Ciesielski's write-up of the meeting covered just one typed page (it appears in Appendix One). No formal questionnaire was used—nor was there one that could have been used. Although the CDC had a questionnaire to help determine how persons with AIDS might have become infected, there was no equivalent survey to discover how a person with AIDS might have infected others. (The CDC has since developed a standard questionnaire to administer to health care workers implicated in HIV transmission.) The greatest weakness was that although Ciesielski was herself a medical doctor, she was no dentist. Ciesielski, wisely, had conferred with CDC dentists prior to the interview and did later show Bergalis's dental records to another dentist to check their quality. But if a dental investigator had been present at the Acer interview, the CDC might have been able to collect more detailed information about his practice (and in particular about his infection control practices and self-injuries).

CDC officials regret not obtaining more information from Acer, but they should hardly be blamed for this omission. Remember, by the early 1990s there were over twelve thousand U.S. AIDS cases initially reported as having unidentified risk factors; several thousand of these were being more or less actively investigated. At the time, Bergalis's case was intriguing but hardly unique. Moreover, because no health care worker had yet been implicated in transmitting HIV to a patient, the CDC had no special reason to believe that it had happened here. As Jaffe explained it,

> The reason that there wasn't a dentist present when we investigated was because at the time it was felt quite unlikely that [Acer] was the source. He was being interviewed with the idea that he would be eliminated as the source of infection. The investigation concentrated on more likely sources.[20]

Moreover, Ciesielski had no way to know that she would be unable to meet again with Acer and a CDC dental expert, if this proved to be necessary. (A confession: Ciesielski has reminded me that I brought no doctor along when I interviewed her!) Ciesielski did have the presence of mind—and the good fortune—to collect blood samples. As we shall see in the next chapter, these samples had the potential to provide the only direct physical evidence that Acer had infected Bergalis.

Ciesielski was not able, for reasons of confidentiality, to ask whether Acer recalled treating Bergalis, although there is no particular reason to think he would have remembered much if asked. Acer had provided dental care to Bergalis six times between November 1987 and June 1989, with the treatment including one examination, two tooth cleanings (prophylaxis), two cosmetic bondings, and one extraction of two molars.[21] None of these treatments had been noteworthy at the time. When Ciesielski showed Bergalis's dental records to another dentist (who did not know the identity of either Bergalis or Acer), this dentist "told us there was no indication from the record that anything unusual had happened, and that in general, he had been impressed with the documentation in [Acer's] charts."[22]

In the following months Economou and Ciesielski devoted a large block of their time to the Bergalis case. The two investigators interviewed and reinterviewed Bergalis, her friends, and her family in an attempt to discover how she might have become infected. This inquiry did not fully exonerate Bergalis, nor did it reject her claims. Economou and Ciesielski were still not completely convinced that they had obtained the entire truth from Bergalis.

For example, the CDC case notes taken from Bergalis's medical records while she was in college suggested a couple of potential concerns. In October 1987, the university infirmary noted that she was seen for genital itching and discharge; at that time she had also denied being sexually active.[23] In January 1988 she visited the university mental health clinic. According to the infirmary's mental health worker, Bergalis came in after her "boyfriend of two years broke up with her. She was upset because he just wanted to kiss her—doesn't want to be sexually involved. She asked boyfriend if he was gay or had a disease and 'he couldn't handle it.'"[24]

The CDC notes indicate further that "it was the impression of her friends that [Bergalis] had sex, most certainly with boyfriend #1, and probably with others, although names were not specified."[25] These statements from Bergalis's peers were, of course, high on speculation and low on documentation; her friends did not really know whether she had had sexual relationships, but they would not have been terribly surprised if she had. In addition, the investigators were not convinced that they had spoken to all the right people. As the investigators summarized it,

> The only friends we could speak to were friends [Bergalis] gave us permission to, and they had all been forewarned by the case that we would be calling. We believe that the case is concerned that, if she tells us her health risk, her mother would find out because she works in a neighboring health department where there is frequent communication. There is reason to believe that the patient believes there would be serious negative impact if her mother believed she participated in any risky behaviors. . . .
> [Bergalis has been] Sexually active (we believe).[26]

Yet by then Bergalis had already conceded as much. While continuing to maintain that she was a virgin, she gradually revealed to Economou and Ciesielski that she had had some sexual contact—but not intercourse—with two former boyfriends. Both individuals were located (one lived in South America) and tested for HIV. Neither tested positive. Even more intriguing was the fact that no one in

Bergalis's circle of friends or acquaintances apparently had HIV. Although HIV is not spread by social contact, it so happens that it tends to cluster within certain social groups that engage in risky behaviors.

(Later, in a videotaped court deposition, Bergalis admitted that she had had some sexual contact with at least one of the two former boyfriends. The *60 Minutes* episode broadcast clips from these tapes as if to demonstrate that Bergalis was more sexually experienced than she had declared and that the CDC had not conducted a thorough investigation of her. Neither innuendo is true. The CDC investigators were well aware of these incidents. Besides, the important thing is that the CDC had contacted the relevant individuals and found that they did not have HIV.)

The investigation was further complicated by Bergalis's relations with her family. Perhaps unavoidably, working with Bergalis's family was difficult for Ciesielski and Economou, and relations were strained. After all, Bergalis's parents wanted to believe that their daughter had not engaged in sexual behavior that put her at risk of contracting HIV, while the investigators had to presume that she probably had. As a result, it was easy for the parents to view the repeated interviewing as an outrage, while the investigators knew that sometimes information was picked up on subsequent interviews that had been omitted from earlier ones.

The strain showed most clearly when other members of the Bergalis family were investigated. If Bergalis truly had contracted HIV in some novel way, then it was possible that she had infected other family members or had been infected by them. (Although there were no documented cases of HIV transmission through casual contact such as in a household setting, it was not entirely inconceivable.) If someone else in the Bergalis family was infected, then perhaps this would provide some clues about how Bergalis herself had contracted HIV. And if no other Bergalis family member tested HIV positive, then Economou at least would be able to rule out certain sources of infection.

Although many families in this situation would probably be eager to submit to blood testing (as Economou noted the Bergalises initially were) both in order to help surveillance officers unravel the mysteries of transmission and to ensure their own well-being, there are also deep-seated sexual taboos that could cause some reluctance. Since HIV is often spread through sexual contact, Economou's request that family members be tested might be construed as an implied accusation that they had committed incest with Bergalis. This accusation is so heinous that innocent and guilty alike might refuse to cooperate with anyone who made it. If another family member did test positive, many people might jump to the conclusion that incest had occurred. This conclusion, of course, would not necessarily be justified; both persons could have contracted the virus from a third source. But the moral judgments of acquaintances and neighbors need not reflect the epidemiological evidence of the case.

While the members of the Bergalis family agreed during their initial interviews to be tested for HIV, Kimberly's father George had not actually come forward for the test. To the father, the delay had simply been a matter of procrastination; he, after all, had no risk factors. But to the surveillance officers, this delay might indicate that the father was worried that the test would incriminate him. When they raised this concern, the Bergalis family was understandably outraged. Mr. Bergalis promptly took the test; the results which demonstrated that Mr. Bergalis was not infected did little to reduce the family's anger.[27] The Bergalis family insisted that the bureaucrats' investigation needed to be more sensitive.

Relations worsened as the investigation continued. A CDC investigator noted that "though initially cooperative, [Bergalis's] mother is now very upset with the investigation and has informed the local health department through an intermediary that we are to leave the family alone as they are being harassed."[28] The family could not help but conclude that investigators thought that Kimberly was lying. These investigators could not help but wonder if she was; it was their job to wonder.

Should Economou and Ciesielski simply have accepted Bergalis's claims? If so, then should surveillance officers believe all NIR claims? Perhaps—but then our understanding of the epidemiology of AIDS would be much weaker because the number of unresolved NIR cases would probably be much larger. Alternately, should the surveillance officers believe no NIR claims unless they can be independently verified? Perhaps—but then the expense and intrusiveness of AIDS investigations would increase substantially. A final possibility is that investigators like Ciesielski and Economou should use their best judgment to decide which claims are likely to be true and which need further investigation. This, indeed, is what they did.

Economou and Ciesielski, in other words, used "bureaucratic discretion" in performing their jobs. Bureaucratic discretion has always been controversial in the United States, where suspicion of and hostility toward government have played a strong role in our historical development. The view that bureaucrats would act capriciously and irresponsibly unless they were given strict orders has motivated recurring actions to limit bureaucratic autonomy.[29] American bureaucrats have thus tended to "go by the book" in performing their duties.[30]

Yet going by the book has its own disadvantages. While it increases consistency in bureaucratic behavior, it also discourages officials from responding appropriately to particular circumstances. The recent trend toward "reinventing government," in fact, is mainly an attempt to allow bureaucrats to use their own judgment in doing their jobs, rather than simply applying formal rules.[31] Although this trend has much intuitive appeal—won't civil servants make better decisions if given the power to do so?—this reinvention will not inevitably become widely adopted. What one bureaucrat may see as good judgment will undoubtedly be viewed by others as arbitrary action. Firmness can be seen as ruthlessness, for example, compassion as weakness, and discretion as arbitrariness.

In this case, the surveillance officers have been variously charged with investigating Bergalis too harshly and too gently. Bergalis's family and Kimberly herself judged the inquiry to be really an inquisition. She testified, "It was hard. I felt like they thought I was lying. You know . . . they came in and just found out everything about me, kind of like an invasion of my privacy. These were things that . . . I cherished, things I've done with my friends. . . . It was hard."[32] According to George Bergalis, "the investigators believed her but didn't *want* to believe her." In the parents' eyes, Economou and Ciesielski did not want the truth; they wanted Kimberly to change her story to confess to some risky behavior. If she did, then the whole issue would just go away.[33]

Yet other critics of the CDC—in particular, Stephen Barr and CBS's *60 Minutes* program—concluded that it had not investigated Bergalis thoroughly enough.[34] According to Barr, the "case against Acer is, at best, astonishingly circumstantial. Some of those who blamed Acer for their fatal illness had other clear risk factors that the health officials overlooked; the rest appear to have been less than forthcoming about their personal lives."[35]

On this point surely Bergalis was right and Barr was wrong. The investigators conducted a highly invasive investigation into Bergalis's life. They had to if they were to verify that she had not engaged in any risky behaviors. No important stones were left unturned. We can be sure of this for two reasons. First, the CDC was aware of *all* the allegations raised in the CBS report and in Barr's articles, and it has rebutted them point by point.[36] Furthermore, those who stood to gain financially by showing that Bergalis and the other patients contracted HIV outside the dental clinic have been unable to build a persuasive case. None of the lawsuits between the patients and Acer's estate or insurance companies has gone to court; all have been settled with the patients receiving substantial monetary awards.

Did Economou and Ciesielski properly balance the desire of the Bergalis family to be treated with dignity and the need for the public health authorities (and the public at large) to learn from whom she had contracted HIV? It is an understatement to suggest that opinions vary on this point. The investigators might argue that their primary responsibility is for *public* health; if private feelings were hurt in this case, so be it. The Bergalis family would argue, in contrast, that they were needlessly hurt and that they had served public health by telling the truth. Both sides, to be sure, have merit. Let us not judge who is right but instead consider how the investigation might have been conducted to satisfy both sides better.

The main problem is that the investigators and Bergalis came to believe that they were opponents rather than allies. The Bergalis family believed that the HRS and the CDC were out to get them; the surveillance officers apparently worked on the assumption that Bergalis was trying to fool them. This conflict need not have existed. The health officials could perhaps have convinced the Bergalis family that they both had a common interest in discovering the real source of Bergalis's infection. How might this have been done?

The HRS and CDC might have started by providing the family with more information about the extraordinary stakes at work in this case. The health officials undoubtedly told the Bergalis family that no health care worker had ever been shown to have infected a patient with HIV—although the CDC knew that this *could* happen. The CDC officials must also have understood that this case would potentially receive extraordinary publicity—just as there had been so much press when Rock Hudson developed AIDS or Ryan White attempted to attend a public school while infected.

This, then, is where the common interest existed. The health officials might have told Bergalis, "Yours is truly a tragedy. We believe you when you say that your only potential exposure to HIV was your dentist. But many people will believe neither you for saying this nor us for reporting it. These people will do everything to show that we are wrong. It is therefore absolutely essential *for both of us* that we identify all possible sources of infection so that we can rule them out."

This statement of common interest would have been neither hypocritical nor manipulative. Hindsight shows it to have been entirely true. Many people *did* try to discredit Bergalis's account. Many people *did* try to show that the CDC had bungled the investigation. If it was discovered that Bergalis had lied about her behavioral risks, she and the CDC would have been publicly humiliated. In the end, the reputations of Bergalis and the CDC were justified because they both *had* told the truth.

Let us return for a moment to the question of whether there was any sympathetic way for the CDC to learn whether incest had been the source of Bergalis's infection. By focusing on their common interests, the health officials might have made the case that "others will make this horrid accusation. We must rule it out by testing all family members."

The suggestion that the investigation would have gone more smoothly and caused less pain if the CDC had identified a common interest with the Bergalis family is not entirely hypothetical. In some ways, this was the approach adopted by her attorney, Robert Montgomery (of the law firm of Montgomery and Larmoyeux, which represented Bergalis in her lawsuits against Acer's estate). In their first meeting, Montgomery laid out some of the difficult issues Bergalis would face:

> Most people think every person who gets AIDS is bad. They must have done something wrong or they wouldn't have gotten "God's curse." . . .
> I want you to know, Kim, I accept that you got AIDS from your dentist. But most people, nearly everyone, will not believe that. . . That [you contracted HIV through risky behavior is] what most people will think about you, Kim. . . .
> [T]he public media will eventually get involved, and they have a way of uncovering nearly everything, particularly things you might not want publicized. . . . And if the media finds out [about this case], they will swarm your house. . . . It's not a pleasant experience. . . .

I will try to protect your health, but I can't . . . try the case without your input. It may be physically debilitating at times, and you, your folks, perhaps your doctors, must decide if you wish to—if you *can* go through that.[37]

While public health officials could learn some lessons about dealing with such cases by watching Montgomery's firm, the lessons are not perfect. Montgomery, after all, was able to do "the little things" to help Bergalis feel better—such as provide her with a car and give her money. (Barr reports that Montgomery gave Bergalis an envelope containing $5,000 in $100 bills and a note saying, "Everything's going to be OK. We'll take care of you. This is yours—a gift from your friend, Bob Montgomery."[38]) Public health officials, meanwhile, cannot even buy someone lunch while on the job. (Montgomery did not exactly go by the book himself. The Florida bar's guidelines declare, "A lawyer shall not provide financial assistance to a client in connection with pending or contemplated litigation." Montgomery acknowledges violating this code but states that "I didn't give a damn in this case."[39])

The second, more important limit is that Montgomery was an advocate for Bergalis; his sole obligation was to represent Bergalis in her lawsuits in the most effective way possible. But what if his firm had come across some truly incriminating information about Bergalis? Health officials would have had to release this information; legal advisers would not. No matter what, Montgomery and Bergalis had reason to show that she had been infected by the dentist, while the health officials ultimately had to be a judge and jury willing to determine whether Acer had infected her or not.

So we cannot fool ourselves into thinking that the Bergalis family and the health officials had perfectly matching interests. Only the Bergalis family could say, "Our daughter is dying. Is yours?" But this difference existed no matter what the CDC did. With enough skill and sensitivity—a high expectation, to be sure—the health officials might have been able to identify and explain the concerns they did share with Bergalis. They probably would have come to the same conclusions, but they also might have spread less pain along the way.

THE CDC ANNOUNCEMENT

It was becoming increasingly clear during the spring and summer that Kimberly Bergalis was a most unusual AIDS case. While Ciesielski and

Economou were investigating Bergalis in Florida, scientists at the CDC headquarters in Atlanta and the Los Alamos National Laboratory in New Mexico were conducting genetic analyses of the blood specimens given by Bergalis and Acer. These analyses showed that the viruses within these two persons were quite similar, suggesting that they had a common source of infection. This finding, together with failure to identify other risk factors for Bergalis, implied that Acer had infected Bergalis.

As the evidence that Acer had infected Bergalis built up from the CDC's field and lab investigations, CDC officials became increasingly worried about how to release this news. They correctly surmised that because this would be the first known case of a health care worker transmitting HIV to a patient, their announcement would be highly visible and heavily scrutinized. If they announced that a dentist had transmitted HIV to a patient—and later had to retract this announcement—then they were sure to be blamed for acting prematurely and thus creating needless public hysteria. (Indeed, medical organizations generally did criticize the CDC for announcing a "possible transmission" rather than waiting until it had a "definite transmission." But it is worth remembering that blood banks had made similar, ill-advised criticisms of the CDC early in the AIDS epidemic.) Yet they also knew that if they delayed publication of this case they would be condemned for withholding essential public health information.

The responsibility for making the decision to publish or to wait rested mainly on the shoulders of Harold Jaffe, now deputy director for science in the CDC's Division of HIV/AIDS, and James Curran, that division's director. Curran, Jaffe, and the others involved in the investigation did not have the luxury to prepare the article about Kimberly Bergalis and David Acer, always called "Patient A" and the "Florida dentist" by the CDC, slowly and deliberately. By July 1990, rumors were already swirling around the health offices in Atlanta and Florida about the Acer case. In the rush to release its study, the CDC (together with the HRS) revised article drafts up until almost the last minute.

While Jaffe, Ciesielski, and Gerald Myers (the scientist who compared the HIV in the blood samples given by Acer and Bergalis) were finalizing the scientific revisions, Curran and Florida officials, especially John Witte, the assistant health officer for disease control and AIDS prevention for the HRS, and Dorothy Miller, the senior attorney for that division, were resolving the legal ones. The most important problem involved confidentiality. The CDC, of course, was not about to disclose the names of the persons involved in the investigation. Yet Witte and Miller nonetheless argued that the CDC's draft article

> permits breach of confidentiality and represents a possible violation of Florida law. [Florida's Omnibus AIDS Law of 1988 protected the confidentiality and work rights of all those in Florida with AIDS.] The case report contains identifiers that may allow the patient to recognize herself, and she in turn would be able to identify the dentist. . . . Advocacy groups and providers may characterize this as a betrayal of our guarantee of confidentiality and counsel their constituents to avoid testing and withhold reporting of additional cases. Moreover, voluntary patient participation in future research could be hampered despite assurances of confidentiality such as those given to the dentist and to the patient in the investigation of this case.[40]

Witte and Miller conceded that violations of confidentiality might be warranted if the information was necessary to demonstrate that HIV had been transmitted within a dental clinic or to prevent imminent danger to the public. But in this case, these conditions did not exist: the dentist was no longer in practice, and the patient's personal characteristics (Bergalis's age, gender, or residence) were irrelevant to the report. Curran revised the report to meet these objections.

This made sense. The CDC and those whom it investigates have a common interest in protecting confidentiality. The subjects of the inquiries need to be confident that their HIV status will not become public (unless they choose to make it so). Although it is illegal to discriminate against persons with AIDS, it is nevertheless the sad fact that many individuals with HIV have reason to fear the reaction of their family, friends, and associates. From the perspective of the HIV-positive individual, public disclosure should take place only at the time and place of that person's choosing.

In the view of public health officials, protection of individual confidentiality is also essential if they are to be able to conduct AIDS surveillance. Unless individuals can be guaranteed that their confidentiality will be protected, they will have strong reasons not to cooperate in the investigation. Yet as we have seen in the Bergalis case, AIDS surveillance can be difficult even when individuals do cooperate. Without this cooperation, reliable surveillance would be almost hopeless. The CDC could not have told Bergalis that Acer had infected her or inform Acer that he had transmitted HIV to Bergalis without violating confidentiality. And once such information is revealed, in a moment the whole world can know.

The CDC chose the accurately but unpleasantly titled *Morbidity and Mortality Weekly Report* (the *MMWR*) in which to make its announcement. The *MMWR*, the house publication of the CDC, carries the latest illness statistics, articles about interesting cases, and other material of concern to health officials. Although articles submitted to the *MMWR* are not subject to peer review by other scientists (as is standard procedure for other respected medical journals) and hence they are considered "provisional," its reports do receive substantial scrutiny from CDC officials themselves. The article announcing the "Possible Transmission of HIV to a Patient During an Invasive Dental Procedure," published on July 27, 1990, certainly received such scrutiny.[41] As a result, it is a model of scientific and public health restraint. It described only the most relevant details of the field and lab investigations. Its conclusion that a dentist had possibly infected a patient while providing dental care was based on three considerations.

First, the patient had had an invasive procedure performed by a dentist with AIDS, and such procedures had been associated with transmission of hepatitis B virus, another bloodborne pathogen, to patients. Second, the CDC's field investigation did not identify any other risk factors or behaviors that may have placed the woman at risk for HIV infection. Third, the viral DNA sequences of the patient and the dentist were closely related.[42] The CDC also reported, however, that this evidence was not foolproof. In particular, the CDC acknowledged that "it is uncertain whether the patient was exposed to the dentist's blood during the [tooth] extraction procedure." Moreover, it noted that "although multiple interviews with this patient and other persons did not identify any established risk factors for HIV infection, such risk factors involve sensitive personal behaviors that may not always be revealed during interviews." Finally, the CDC reported that the "use of DNA sequencing for this purpose is new . . . and the quantitative criteria for determining epidemiologic linkage based on HIV sequences are just now being developed."[43] In other words, the CDC told the world, We think it happened, but we are not sure.

The CDC did not call Bergalis before releasing the *MMWR*. Instead, Bergalis first heard the word that night on the *NBC Nightly*

News, when Jane Pauley announced that the CDC had just released a report indicating that a dentist in Florida had apparently transmitted HIV to a young woman while providing her dental care. This CDC report—covered that evening by all three major television networks—outraged Bergalis. The standards of Florida and the CDC regarding confidentiality, designed to protect those they investigated, provided little solace to Bergalis—or Economou, for that matter. Although Bergalis had little doubt that the CDC report was referring to her, she called Economou shortly after watching the NBC news to confirm her suspicions. When Bergalis reached Economou, Nikki asked if she could return the call. After forty-five minutes—presumably as Economou was trying to get advice about what to do—Nikki called back. She told Bergalis something like "You know I can't tell you if you are the person. . . . Assuming you are this person, assuming that it was the dentist . . . things are pretty hectic up in Atlanta at the CDC, and the phones were ringing off the wall."[44]

If Economou did not know exactly how to handle Bergalis's questions, the CDC knew that its announcement meant that a great number of questions would have to be answered. In preparation for this, Jaffe issued his staff "briefing notes" as well as practice questions and answers pending the release of the *MMWR.* These notes had the joint goal of calming the public and convincing it that the CDC knew what it was doing. The notes stated that "if the present case does represent [HIV] transmission [from health care worker to patient during treatment], it was not unanticipated."[45] The CDC had already written in 1987 that "although transmission of HIV from infected health care workers to patients has not been reported, transmission during invasive procedures remains a possibility" and that numerous guidelines issued by the CDC since 1982 had sought to minimize that possibility.[46] It did concede, however, that the CDC was again reviewing its guidelines.

While the question and answer section of this memo mainly reiterated CDC findings and policy (for example, the CDC did not recommend that all health care workers be tested for HIV; restrictions on HIV-positive health care workers should be made on a case-by-case basis; health care workers should follow CDC guidelines to reduce risks of transmission; and so on), one question and answer would prove especially troublesome for those working on this issue:

Q: Would you let your spouse/child/yourself undergo an invasive procedure by an HIV-infected health care worker?

A: My personal feelings are not important in answering this question. However . . . more than half of the respondents [of a nationwide survey] felt that dentists and surgeons should not be allowed to continue working if they are infected with HIV. This survey . . . reflects concern not necessarily based on fact.[47]

This concern was certainly Bergalis's. She and her family were understandably bitter that the CDC had not seemed to consider her feelings and say to her, "Yes, you were right. Your dentist infected you with HIV." (Jaffe insists that they very much wanted to inform her but were told by HRS officials in Florida that this was not legal. Florida officials, for their part, had tried to persuade Acer to let them notify Bergalis that he was the likely source of infection, but Acer refused.) It was only natural for Bergalis to wish for a personal response. But there are both good and legal reasons why the CDC did not tell her. Legally, the HRS—and by implication, the CDC—was bound to protect patient confidentiality. Whether or not we agree with the law, do we really want our governmental agencies to break it whenever some people see fit? (It is noteworthy that Bergalis also tried to protect her anonymity. Her lawsuit against the Acer estate was originally filed under the initials *K. B. v. D. A.* Only after it became obvious that the media would discover whose initials these were did Bergalis herself decide to reveal her identity.) Moreover, telling a person from whom they contracted HIV is likely to lead to retaliations—perhaps lawful, perhaps violent—against that person. Do we really want our public health agencies to provoke this vengeance?

WERE OTHER PATIENTS AT RISK?

Horrible possibilities were now on the health officials' minds. If Acer had infected Bergalis, then had he also infected other patients? If a single patient had contracted HIV in a medical setting, then would patients in other medical settings also start claiming that their health care provider had infected them? Again, Florida's confidentiality laws slowed the investigation at this critical juncture. The CDC could not, without Acer's consent, contact his former patients or staff. Until Acer gave this consent, public health officials could not bring his patients in for interviews and blood tests.

For two hours on Friday night, August 10, 1990, HRS officials James Howell (Economou's boss), Spencer Lieb, and Laurel Hopper (an HRS attorney) met with Acer, his parents and brother, and his attorney Deborah Sawyer to persuade the dentist to allow the HRS to contact his patients. Acer was reluctant to do so; but by the end of the meeting promised to cooperate.

A second brief meeting—and a real breakthrough—came two weeks later, when Acer signed an "Authorization for Release of Patient Names."[48] This meant that Acer (or, actually, his attorney Sawyer) would grant the HRS access to the names and addresses of any patient he had treated after 1983. (Although Acer had already turned over the records he possessed to Ciesielski and Economou, this release meant that HRS could obtain names and addresses from other sources.) Still, this release placed strict limits on the investigators. The patients' dental records could not be disclosed to the HRS; indeed, Florida law specifically prohibited such disclosure.[49] Moreover, in contacting the patients to alert them to the possibility that they might have been exposed to HIV, the investigators could not reveal Acer's name, his HIV status, or even use the terms "health care provider" or "dentist" in describing the potential source of exposure. This protection of Acer's privacy was also mandated by Florida law.[50] Finally, the release stated that Acer's consent should not be construed as an admission that he had infected anyone with HIV.

To prepare for meeting Acer's patients, the HRS drafted mock interviews for its surveillance officers to help them inform the patients, without mentioning Acer, that they might have been exposed to HIV. These mock interviews are, at best, strained. In one prescient scenario, a sixty-two-year-old female who is married with children and grandchildren is interviewed in the presence of her husband, who will not leave the room.

OFFICER: Mrs. Smith, the reason I am here is to inform you that the HRS has knowledge of your possible exposure to the virus that causes AIDS. . . .

PATIENT: How could I have been exposed? I have never had sex with anyone but my husband and I don't do drugs and, as my husband said, I have never had a blood transfusion. My husband has been impotent for six years so how could I be exposed?

OFFICER: I am relatively sure there is nothing to worry about but, as I stated earlier, I have knowledge of your possible exposure, and because of confidentiality laws I am not at liberty to disclose who [may have exposed you] or how you may have been exposed.[51]

The biggest breakthrough for the HRS came when Acer agreed to publish a letter to his patients urging them to be tested for HIV. Shortly before he died, Acer asked Sawyer to help him write this letter. Sawyer wrote several drafts and showed them to Howell and Acer, who signed the final version on August 31. Acer died on September 3, and the letter was subsequently published as a paid advertisement (so it would be printed without editing) in the local newspaper on Thursday and Friday, September 6 and 7, 1990. Although it is difficult to know whether this letter shows Acer's true sentiments or the advice of his legal counsel, the letter states that:

I am David J. Acer, and I have AIDS. . . . I am writing this letter because I am concerned that with the recent news regarding me in the local media, you are afraid that you may have been infected with the disease commonly known as AIDS. I want to try to reassure you that it is unlikely you have been infected with the disease from me, and to urge you to seek the free testing and counseling that is available from your local health department. . . .

I want each of you to understand that when I became aware that I had tested positive for the HIV virus (AIDS), I consulted with medical experts on whether I should continue practicing dentistry. . . . The experts advised me that as long as I followed the guidelines promulgated by the [CDC] for health care providers who were infected with HIV (AIDS), that I could safely continue to practice as a dentist, and that I would not infect my patients. I reviewed the CDC guidelines and strictly adhered to them. . . .

It is with great sorrow and some surprise that I read that I am accused of transmitting the HIV virus (AIDS) to one of my patients. I do not understand how such a thing could have happened, and I do not believe that it did happen. . . . If the CDC had advised me to stop practicing because the guidelines were not safe, I would have immediately done so. However, it is my belief that the CDC would never issue guidelines that would put patients and health care workers at risk in transmitting this disease.

However, you understandably are frightened. For your peace of mind, I suggest that you please contact the local health department for free testing and counseling. . . . If the CDC guidelines are valid, you should not be infected. . . .

Finally, please try to understand. I am a gentle man, and I would never intentionally expose anyone to this disease. I have cared for people all my life, and to infect anyone with this disease would be contrary to everything I have stood for. I am sorry if this news story has caused you fear and worry.

This remarkable letter provided opportunities, puzzles, and problems for the CDC. Most helpfully, it finally allowed the CDC to contact and test Acer's other patients. Without this permission, it is unlikely that many patients would ever have come in for testing.

The letter also perplexed the investigators, however. Had Acer truly "reviewed the CDC guidelines and strictly adhered to them," and if so, how had infection occurred? Was Acer really a "gentle man [who] would never intentionally expose anyone to this disease"? To answer these questions would surely require additional investigation.

The final issues were even more problematic. Had the CDC misled the medical community as well as the general public about the safety of the health care system? Were the CDC guidelines themselves at fault? Resolving these matters would trouble CDC officials throughout the coming years.

Once Acer had written his open letter and had given the HRS permission to contact his former patients, the investigators moved swiftly to identify these patients and encourage them to come in for HIV tests. As Acer's letter received widespread publicity, many of his patients heard about the case and offered themselves for testing. But because CDC and HRS officials viewed it essential to reach as many patients as possible in order to know whether Acer had infected anyone else, they also conducted an aggressive outreach program. Unfortunately, it was not clear how many patients Acer had actually treated after he had HIV (although HRS officials guessed that it was probably between 2,400 and 2,700). Robert Scott, the HRS official leading this outreach effort, had already obtained a list of 128 patients from the records Acer had kept at home. Now he persuaded CIGNA, the health insurance company that had referred many of its customers to Acer, to share its list; over 2,000 names were obtained in this way. But CIGNA, although willing to share its referral lists, did not know which of its customers had actually used Acer's services. To identify the actual patients, Scott then contacted other local dentists accepting CIGNA customers (as well as other dentists in the area) to see whether Acer's patients had sought treatment with them after Acer retired.

The day Acer's letter was published—September 6—the district health office began offering HIV testing and counseling to those former patients who came in to learn whether they had been infected.

About 800 patients came in of their own accord. This initial surge of testing diminished by November, at which point the HRS sent nearly 2,000 certified letters to patients who had not yet come in. This letter convinced another 141 patients to step forward. (The response is a reminder of how mobile U.S. residents are—or how unwilling to receive official mail: almost 800 of the certified letters were returned unopened to the HRS.) Ultimately, almost 1,100 of Acer's patients were tested for HIV, with the Palm Beach County health clinic testing (by its count) 953 of them. No one knows how many patients were tested privately and did not report the results to public health officials.

Health officials have found ten of Acer's patients who were infected with HIV. As with Bergalis, Ciesielski and Economou had to conduct investigations of each of these persons to learn how he or she might have been exposed to the virus. Each person had special characteristics that challenged the investigators' surveillance skills. Let us meet these individuals briefly in order to understand some of the difficulties Ciesielski and Economou faced.[52] The names of these patients have never been revealed by the CDC but have become public knowledge through the media.

Patient B, Barbara Webb, seemed remarkably like the hypothetical Mrs. Smith in the HRS practice interviews. A schoolteacher in her sixties, she had visited Acer's office twenty-one times between December 1987 and July 1989 and had received a wide variety of treatments, including four tooth extractions. Ms. Webb had been married for forty years, and her husband was not infected. She denied engaging in behaviors that put her at risk of contracting HIV. Yet the investigation of Webb—who appeared to cooperate fully and willingly with her questioners—exposed two question marks. First, she acknowledged having an extramarital affair in the late 1970s. This affair took place before the breakout of AIDS in the United States, although not before HIV was present; her partner, although presumably at low risk for being infected, was not tested. While there is virtually no chance that Webb could have contracted HIV then, that chance is not quite zero. Second, it is unclear whether Webb received a blood transfusion during surgery she experienced in the early 1980s as someone made a mistake in record keeping then. When Webb entered surgery, blood was checked out for her use, and this blood was never checked back in; this suggests that Webb did receive a transfusion. Yet Webb's hospital charts do not actually show that the transfusion was administered. Once again, however, even if she received a transmission there was only a small likelihood that the blood was infected with HIV. Still, the possibility existed—though it seemed remote—that Webb had been exposed to HIV outside the dental clinic.

The case of Patient C, Richard Driskill, was just as puzzling but for quite different reasons. Driskill, age thirty-one, was married and had been Acer's patient since 1984. He admitted to using cocaine but denied injecting drugs. He also revealed that he had numerous extramarital affairs. He could remember the names of fourteen of his sexual partners since 1978; the CDC was able to locate and test nine of them, and they all tested negative. More troublesome were the many rumors that Driskill had sexual contacts with males and prostitutes. Driskill denied these allegations, and the CDC was unable to prove that Driskill had been exposed to HIV in any of his sexual encounters. Acer had administered a variety of treatments (once again, including a couple of extractions) over the course of Driskill's fourteen visits.

Webb and Driskill had both responded to Acer's open letter and had come to the county clinic for testing, as they had no symptoms leading them to suspect that they might have been infected. Patient D, in contrast, had been identified by the HRS when it compared the list of Acer's patients to the state's AIDS surveillance records. Patient D had been treated by Acer eighteen times between 1985 and 1989. This individual, who already had AIDS, acknowledged having behavioral risk factors and assumed that he had contracted HIV through these behaviors. As the CDC eventually concluded that he had not been infected by Acer, there was little popular interest in his story. Patient D's name thus has not become public knowledge.

Patient E, Lisa Shoemaker, had come to Florida in the summer of 1988 while she was working for the circus. Between June and December of that year she visited Acer's office fourteen times for examinations, cleanings, a filling, and two root canals, among other treatments. Like Patient D, she also believed originally that she had contracted HIV through her own sexual behavior. Shoemaker and her boyfriend had been tested for HIV in October 1988 (more than a year before Bergalis was diagnosed) after she discovered that her boyfriend was bisexual. At that time both she and her boyfriend tested negative. Still worried, they were both tested again in December 1988. At that point, she tested positive for the virus—but he did not. Still, assuming that somehow her boyfriend had given her the virus, she broke up with him and moved back to her parents' home in Michigan.

In December 1990, responding to national publicity about the case, Shoemaker called the CDC and announced that she had been one of Acer's patients. After confirming this, Ciesielski questioned her, with Shoemaker's attorney present for the entire interview. Shoemaker could name ten sexual partners since 1978. Two of these contacts had died (but not from AIDS), and they were not known to have been at risk for HIV. The other eight partners were located and tested, and one tested HIV positive.

This person was Patient F, the boyfriend whom Shoemaker suspected of infecting her. Patient F, as it turns out, had also been one of Acer's patients while Shoemaker and he were in Florida. The available records showed that Patient F had visited Acer only once, although he remembered five or six visits for routine checkups, fillings, and a root canal. Patient F did have behavioral risk factors, as Shoemaker herself had already observed. Yet Patient F tested negative for HIV both times he went in for blood tests with Shoemaker. It wasn't until two years after Shoemaker had tested positive for HIV—two years after the two had last had sexual contact—that Patient F was diagnosed as HIV positive. Patient F did have symptoms—sore throat, headache, and diarrhea, among others—consistent with the early stages of HIV infection in September 1989; these symptoms often develop within the first three months after infection. Patient F's symptoms occurred about one year after his last dental appointment with Acer and last sexual contact with Shoemaker. This meant that he had not infected Shoemaker nor been infected by her. As with Patient D, Patient F's name has not become public knowledge because the CDC concluded that Acer had not infected him.

Patient G, John Yecs, was an alcoholic in his thirties. The drug and alcohol rehabilitation facility at which he was receiving treatment took him to Acer a couple of times for a root canal and a dental filling. While Yecs admitted to abusing alcohol (and other drugs, such as cocaine), he denied injecting drugs. The CDC's review of his medical records indicated that there was no evidence he had used intravenous drugs since the late 1970s, before the onset of AIDS in the United States. Although it was reported that he had visited prostitutes (and indeed had traded drugs for sex), the CDC could not confirm these reports. (Stephen Barr describes a videotaped deposition in which a prostitute testifies that she saw another prostitute who died from AIDS frequently perform oral sex on Yecs while he was not wearing a condom.[53]) His two confirmed sexual partners both tested negative for HIV. Yecs tested positive for HIV when he attempted to donate blood plasma for a small fee in 1990.

The anonymous patients H and J have acknowledged that they had behavioral risk factors for AIDS, and the CDC has concluded that neither was infected by the dentist.

Patient I, Sherry Johnson, was still in high school when she tested positive for HIV in routine screening when she volunteered for the armed forces. Johnson reported having had sexual contact with six men. Five of these men were identified and tested—all tested negative—but the sixth man could not be located. Johnson claimed that she had only had a single sexual contact with him, however, and that he had used a condom. Only one visit to Acer's office could be documented for Johnson, but she and her family believed that Acer had treated her on three occasions.

Ciesielski and Economou, together with others such as Bob Scott and Ken Bell who helped with the investigation, thus had to discover the most intimate details in the lives of men and women, young and old, married and unmarried, chaste and promiscuous, sober and drunk. Documenting (not surmising) exposure to HIV for any one of these individuals created difficult problems for the investigators; doing so for all of them must certainly have challenged the officers' creativity and persistence. Note, however, that in *none* of the cases could the investigators prove that a patient had been infected by someone other than Acer. While at least some of the patients acknowledged behavioral risk factors (which created the presumption—but not the conclusion—that they had been infected outside the dental clinic), in no case could the investigators be certain that they had found the source of infection. On the other hand, in *no case* could Ciesielski and Economou absolutely rule out the possibility that HIV *had* been contracted from someone other than Acer. While some patients (for example, Bergalis and Webb) seemed unlikely to have been infected by someone other than the dentist, other patients (such as Driskill, Shoemaker, and Yecs) seemed more likely to have contracted the virus through their own behaviors. In other words, Ciesielski and Economou faced the daily reality that their most talented and diligent efforts would not—and could not—provide definitive answers to the question: Who infected these patients?

For these answers, the CDC turned away from its field investigation and toward a genetic one.

CHAPTER THREE

Science
The Genetic Analysis Links Acer
to His Patients

———〰〰———

Good scientists are good detectives. They start with a mystery, develop their leads, collect and examine the evidence, puzzle over its meaning, and then, if they are skilled and lucky, develop enough evidence to convince the jury. The CDC's surveillance officers had identified the prime suspect: David Acer. It was now the scientists' job to do their detective work in determining if he, indeed, was the one.

In the simplest of investigations, the suspect leaves a singularly incriminating mark—say, a fingerprint or signature—for the detectives. But this was not a simple case. The scientists did not only have to ask "Are Acer's 'fingerprints' on the patients?" but also "What exactly is an HIV fingerprint?"

Consider the ordinary fingerprint. It is a valuable tool for identification because each person's is unique and constant. Fingerprints change little over time, and they are virtually perfect at identifying individuals. If a person's fingerprints are on another, we can conclude that the second person has been touched by the first.

HIV, in contrast, is perpetually mutating. This means that within any infected individual, there is a "swarm" of viruses that may differ slightly from each other and that gradually change over time. And because HIV is an infectious disease, each HIV-positive person's viruses are literally related to every other person's, bearing more or less resemblance depending on how closely linked the infections are to each other. Consider the HIV within Tiffany, Steven, and Keisha, the individuals we investigated in the previous chapter. If Steven actually infected both women, their viruses will likely resemble his more closely than they will those in each other. Still, the viruses within Tiffany and Keisha will typically bear a closer resemblance to each other than to a person who had not been infected by Steven. Each infected person has been touched, but the question is by whom?

At the time of the Bergalis investigation, Gerald Myers—director of the HIV Sequence Database at the Los Alamos National Laboratory—and other scientists had already begun to learn how much HIV varies within individuals, among persons known to have a common source of infection, and among persons with only distantly related viruses.[1] This knowledge was developed by comparing the viral DNA in people for whom it was known whether or not they had infected each other. For example, infants who contracted HIV in the womb are certain to have been infected by their mothers and thus to share a closely related virus, while HIV-positive individuals living permanently in different parts of the world are unlikely to have infected each other and so most likely do not carry closely related viruses.

An analogy might clarify this point. We might think of the body as an infinitely complex and varied book of life, with HIV as one of its potential stories. When we write these stories down, we can break them down into smaller units, with chromosomes as the paragraphs, genes as the sentences, and nucleotides—smaller genetic components still—as the words. Like words, the nucleotides can be depicted as a series of letters, with each letter representing a particular chemical component, or "nitrogen base"; the most common letters are A (for adenine), G (guanine), C (cytosine), and U (uracil). The arrangement, or sequence, of these letters "constitutes the unique structural and functional individuality of DNA molecules."[2] The stories in the book of life are determined ultimately by the arrangement of these genetic letters. Small changes in the arrangement of the letters can have a large impact on the meaning of the story.

Myers reasoned that by examining the arrangement of the letters, he could see how much viruses differed from one another. For

Person	Genetic Sequence	Percent Agreement with X, Virus 1		
		X, Virus 2	Y	Z
X, Virus 1	ATAATCCACCTATCCCAGTA	95%	90%	70%
X, Virus 2	ATA**T**TCCACCTATCCCAGTA		85%	65%
Y	AT**T**ATCCACCTATCC**A**AGTA			60%
Z	A**A**AATT**C**C**C**CAAT**T**CCAGT**T**			

Table 3.1. Hypothetical Genetic Sequences in Three Persons' HIV
ᵃBases that differ from Person X, Virus 1 are marked in bold.
Source: The sequence in Virus 1 was taken from David E. Kellog and Shirley Kwok, "Detection of Human Immunodeficiency Virus," in M. A. Innis, D. H. Gelfand, J. Sninsky, and T. J. White, eds., *PCR Protocols: A Guide to Methods and Applications* (New York: Academic Press, 1990), p. 339.

instance, say that we know Person X has infected Person Y with HIV and that neither individual has had contact with Person Z. We now draw two small samples of the virus from X and one from Y and Z and compare them. The genetic sequences from these HIV samples might look something like those shown in Table 3.1. In this illustration, the sequences from the two viruses taken from Person X agree 95 percent of the time (at only one of the twenty locations do the letters differ). The sequences from Person X and Person Y have agreements of 90 and 85 percent. In contrast, Person Z's virus matches the other two individuals' HIV at between 60 and 70 percent of the letters. While the differences in the viruses illustrated here are somewhat larger than in real life, they do show the typical pattern; the DNA sequences of the HIV within a single infected person are typically 95 to 100 percent the same.[3] In general, the similarity among viruses is highest within a single person, somewhat lower for viruses obtained from persons who have a common source of infection, and lowest between persons who did not directly share infections.

Still, it was one thing to discover that cases of HIV known to be related were more similar than cases known to be unrelated; it was wholly another to look at the genetic sequences to determine whether cases of HIV were actually related. This had never been done before. Yet this is exactly what the scientists examining the HIV in Acer, Bergalis, and the others had to do. The critical questions for these scientists were these:

Exactly what portions of the viral story should be examined? How similar did the genetic sequences need to be before one could conclude that Acer had infected his patients? What needed to be done to convince other scientists and the public that these conclusions were correct?

Two issues complicated matters. The scientists were under tremendous pressure to answer the questions quickly, before rumors about the investigations were leaked to the media. And the press was all over this investigation, in part because of the public's tremendous interest in it, in part because certain journalists were well connected to the CDC. (A former editor of the *MMWR* was now a reporter for the *New York Times*, for example, and he had ready access to CDC officials.) In at least one instance, the *Los Angeles Times* announced the results of one patient's genetic analysis before it could be published in the *MMWR*, a move that the leading researcher called "very disturbing and disruptive."[4] The scientists, understandably, did not want the results released until they were confident that they had arrived at the correct ones. And while the media created pressure to answer the questions quickly, the scientific community provided strong incentives to get the answers right.

THE GENETIC SEQUENCING STUDY

Although research on the dentist's patients was being conducted almost continuously from March 1990 through May 1992 (and sporadically after that), it might be helpful to think of the genetic investigation as occurring in five distinct stages.[5] Stage 1 began on March 28, 1990, when Ciesielski collected a blood sample from Bergalis; it ended four months later when the CDC released its report that "the laboratory findings in this investigation indicate possible transmission of HIV" from Acer to Bergalis.[6] Stage 2 began on September 6, 1990, with the publication of Acer's letter to his former patients, encouraging them to come forward for HIV testing. In the following months, four other HIV-infected patients (Barbara Webb, Richard Driskill, Patient D, and Lisa Shoemaker) were identified. This stage ended when the CDC released its report on Webb, Driskill, and Patient D in January 1991.[7] Immediately afterward came Stage 3, in which the CDC analyzed the DNA in Shoemaker, Patient F, and John Yecs; its

June 1991 report announced that Shoemaker and Yecs had also contracted HIV from Acer.[8] In Stage 4, the CDC further refined its genetic investigation of the seven HIV-infected patients already identified.[9] While the article published in May 1992 was declared to have "closed" the Acer case, three other HIV-infected individuals (patients H and J and Sherry Johnson) were later recognized as Acer's patients, and their DNA was analyzed in Stage 5.[10]

Each stage contained three main steps. In the first, CDC researchers selected individuals to include in the study and then took blood samples from them; these individuals included both patients and other HIV-positive individuals to be used as a comparison group. This was usually done in Florida by CDC and HRS field investigators. Next, researchers extracted and sequenced DNA fragments from the blood samples. This step took place primarily in laboratories at the CDC under the direction of CDC scientists. Third, researchers conducted statistical analyses on these genetic sequences to determine their similarity. This step was performed principally by contractors hired by the CDC at the Los Alamos National Laboratory (LANL) in New Mexico.

While the researchers at each site actually performed the work, the decisions about what work should be performed were made cooperatively by those in the field in Florida, at the CDC headquarters in Georgia, in the research lab in New Mexico, and by scientists from Scotland to Stanford. Selecting individuals from whom to collect blood samples was influenced both by what was needed by the LANL analysts and what was available to the Florida investigators. Extracting and sequencing the DNA was determined by what was possible in the labs at the CDC and what was useful for analysis in New Mexico. Scientific research is no longer, if it ever was, simply the solo pursuit of knowledge; it is always and everywhere a team effort.

THE CDC EXTRACTS THE DNA

When the CDC's Carol Ciesielski first interviewed Bergalis on March 28, 1990, she took a sample of Bergalis's blood. The following day, at the conclusion of her interview with Acer, Ciesielski also withdrew three ten-milliliter blood specimens from the dentist. This first step was critically important: these blood samples would become the only evidence directly linking the HIV in Acer and his patients. The blood would not reveal the evidence easily, however. The steps needed to be taken carefully, or they would become missteps. Although she did not know it, there would be no more chances to obtain blood from the dentist. Ciesielski packed the vials and delivered them the next day to Chin-Yih Ou at the CDC labs in Atlanta.

Ou was a pioneer in the microbiology of HIV. While at the CDC in 1988, for example, he directed a study that developed a test to identify HIV in blood, which allowed a quicker diagnosis of individuals than had been available through conventional tests; the conventional tests looked for the antibodies of HIV, and these took up to six months after infection to develop.[11] Ou's CDC lab had extensive experience in using the polymerase chain reaction (PCR) procedure to extract the DNA from HIV and the sequencing kits to determine the order of the bases.

The PCR procedure had revolutionized molecular research. Developed in 1985, PCR by 1990 had already been used in more than six hundred scientific publications involving genetic analyses, diagnosis of inherited disorders, susceptibility to disease, and evolution.[12] PCR is exquisitely sensitive, which is a good thing because HIV can be difficult to detect. It can correctly identify and amplify HIV molecules when they are as scarce as one in ten thousand in blood specimens.[13] This sensitivity also means that PCR is prone to contamination. For PCR to be used successfully, therefore, extreme care has to be taken every step of the way.

Ou's lab accordingly took numerous steps to ensure that the DNA in this study was accurately extracted and sequenced.[14] For example, he used CDC laboratory facilities that were specifically dedicated to PCR but had not previously been used for HIV extraction (to ensure that no stray HIV was lurking around the lab). Vials and laboratory benches were irradiated to destroy other genetic material that might be present. Chemicals used in the process were measured for a single use. Only one blood sample was processed at a time. These steps helped ensure that the HIV was not tainted from other sources.

Ou and his staff also performed several tests to see whether the genetic information had become contaminated during PCR. These tests essentially consisted of dividing each person's blood specimen into two samples and then extracting and sequencing genetic material from each sample. The sequences from each sample were compared with each other as well as other specimens. But because HIV varies within each person, it is not possible to use HIV sequences to confirm that two blood specimens come from the same person. Ou therefore also sequenced the human leukocyte antigen (HLA), which does not vary within an individual. Comparing these HLA sequences allowed Ou to confirm that two specimens came from the same person and differed from the other person.

As yet another check on the quality of the DNA extraction and sequencing, the work of Ou's lab was replicated by Dr. A. J. Leigh Brown and his colleagues at the University of Edinburgh, Scotland. (Leigh Brown was somewhat of a prodigy as a population geneticist, having already received his Ph.D. and been published in *Nature* by the age of twenty-four. He conducted the seminal research that traced the HIV infections in a group of hemophiliacs—the "Edinburgh cohort"—back to a single lot of blood.[15]) This replication was neither easy nor automatic. At the time, federal law prohibited the export of infected fresh blood cells, so Ou could not send the samples directly to Leigh Brown. (This law has since been changed to allow such export for research purposes.) Instead, Ou had the DNA extracted in a different CDC lab (as before, one in which no HIV work had previously been done) by different personnel (who had no other contact with this investigation). The DNA for Acer, Bergalis, and one other HIV-positive person was then shipped to Edinburgh. Leigh Brown was at first unable to reproduce the sequences that Ou had extracted or even to identify the HIV in one of the samples.[16] Even prodigies sometimes need to redo their experiments; after doing so, Leigh Brown informed Ou that their sequences were virtually identical. The PCR procedure and the sequencing had been successfully replicated.

Ou's labs had extracted, and both Ou and Leigh Brown had sequenced, approximately 300 to 350 base "letters" from a particular portion of the "sentence" called the HIV's "envelope" gene. This portion was examined for both theoretical and practical reasons. On the theoretical side, the scientists chose to focus on the parts of the virus that showed the greatest diversity. The logic behind this choice was that as this portion was highly variable, if two individuals had similar sequences they probably had a common source of infection. As a practical matter, most previous studies of HIV infection had also looked at this segment and so more data existed from it.

Examining the genetic sequences within the envelope gene was not the only choice open to the scientists, however. Some observers have suggested that attention should have been focused on the most stable portions of the virus rather than the most variable ones. Their logic was that if these portions differed, this would be strong evidence that the individuals had different sources of infection. In other words, these observers thought that the scientists should not have tested to see whether Acer and his patients had a common virus but to see if they had distinct viruses.[17]

Ou also chose to take multiple samples of the virus from Acer and Bergalis and ultimately from the other patients as well. Recall that a person with HIV is not infected by a single virus but by a swarm of viruses. Thus, a single sample—a single set of sequences—of the virus may or may not accurately represent the genetic variability in an individual's HIV. Ou thus chose to obtain from five to twelve different examples of the genetic sequences from each individual. Together, these multiple sequences were believed to portray more accurately the infections of the dentist and his patients than any single sequence could.

Ou was to make a different decision regarding the extraction and sequencing of DNA from the local controls (LC, as the CDC called the HIV-positive individuals in the study who were not Acer's patients). For each LC, Ou's lab essentially took a single DNA "consensus" sample rather than a set of samples (taking multiple samples was technically challenging). Yet no one really understood what this consensus sequence meant. Was it some kind of statistical average of that person's viral sequences? Or was it a unique specimen from the virus? These questions are important because in examining the sequences of Acer, the patients, and the local controls, the researchers vitally needed to compare apples with apples. Unfortunately, no one knew for certain then what an "apple" was.[18]

LOS ALAMOS NATIONAL LABORATORY ANALYZES THE SEQUENCES

The Sangre de Cristo ("Blood of Christ") mountains are much higher and drier than the beaches of southern Florida or the CDC's Atlanta headquarters. In 1942, J. Robert Oppenheimer, the father of the atom bomb, wanted to locate the labs that would first produce these awful weapons here because the mountains were so remote and beautiful.[19] The Los Alamos National Laboratory (LANL), although still producing deadly research, now also has a more benign task: it is home to the most complete set of HIV sequences (in the GenBank) and some of the most sophisticated genetic analyses in the world.

Los Alamos's place in history is assured and its geographical location sublime. The position of the lab within the government is more puzzling. LANL is a "GOCO"—a government-owned, contractor-operated facility. The University of California is the principal contractor that operates the lab. Even though nuclear weapons research still continues, most of its funding comes from the Department of Energy (not Defense). Its research facilities are now used to create the deadliest weapons as well as to defuse the most lethal virus. Oddly enough, its role in HIV research springs from its capacities in weapons research. The Human Genome Project, a massive study to map the entire set of human DNA (a sequence of approximately three billion base pairs), required the most powerful computers; the weapons labs at LANL, of course, had them.[20]

Gerald Myers came to LANL in 1982 as a Ph.D. biophysicist to work as a consultant to GenBank, the predecessor of the Human Genome Project. As he developed expertise in analyzing genetic sequences, investigators from around the world began sending him their HIV sequences to examine and catalogue. By the time the CDC wanted to compare the viruses of Acer and Bergalis, Myers had the reputation, skills, the database, and the title (as director of the HIV Sequence Database) to make him the natural choice to conduct the analysis. The CDC's Curran and Jaffe consequently asked Myers if he could help them with their investigation.

Myers was naturally inclined to accept the CDC's request. This study was going to be intellectually challenging and publicly significant—and not just because it was potentially the first case of HIV transmission from a health care worker to a patient. The study was also conceptually tied to the dispute between Robert Gallo and Luc Montagnier over the discovery of HIV. Gallo claimed to have discovered the cause of AIDS by isolating a virus (he labeled it HTLV-III) a year after Montagnier's lab had isolated a virtually identical virus (labeled LAV). At the time, Gallo had tried to argue that it was possible that two unrelated cases of HIV could look nearly identical by chance; this argument bolstered his claim that he and Montagnier had independently discovered the virus. But if Gallo's argument were true, then a close similarity in the viruses of Acer and Bergalis could also be merely luck and would not imply that Bergalis had been infected by her dentist.[21] Myers was convinced otherwise: just days after President Reagan and the French prime minister had jointly announced that the Americans and the French shared credit for the discovery of HIV, Myers wrote in a confidential memo that this announcement perpetrated a "double fraud." The French, not Gallo, had identified the virus. As Myers wrote, "I suggest that we have paid for this deception in more than the usual ways. Scientific fraudulence always costs humanity . . . but here we have been additionally misdirected with regard to the extent of variation of the virus, which we can ill afford."[22]

Myers's willingness to do the study had little to do with what his lab could afford, even though he worked on "soft money." Like many scientific researchers, Myers was neither a tenured academic nor a bureaucrat. While he received virtually all his funding from the government, he was not guaranteed a salary or a job in perpetuity. Each year he had to bring funded projects into his lab or there would be no lab, no research, and no job. This study would bring in no money, at least not at first. (As his work on this project expanded, Myers eventually received a small contract with the CDC to ensure that his other projects would not be neglected. The initial contract was for the princely sum of $13,376.[23]) Still, his main funding agency, the National Institutes of Health, agreed that Myers's participation in the CDC's study would contribute to NIH's goals and so allowed him to proceed without CDC funding.[24]

Regarding money: even though the Los Alamos labs are located near heaven, their facilities look closer to bargain basement. At the time of the Bergalis study, Myers worked in what might be called a "single wide" mobile home; its main furnishings were computer terminals and stacks of printouts. Myers conducted the genetic analysis himself in the beginning but was joined shortly afterward by Bette Korber, a Ph.D. chemist from Cal Tech, for the rest of the investigation.

The virus had been converted from life (the viral DNA) into data (long strings of letters and symbols in a computer file) by the time Myers received them. Over the next two weeks Myers would subject these data to a wide variety of analytical techniques.[25] The first test Myers conducted involved an exceedingly powerful and sophisticated tool: the expert human mind. Before crunching the data, he looked at them. While the data—line after line of letters depicting the DNA bases—looked to my eyes like the result of a monkey at the keyboard, Myers almost immediately saw patterns that would convince him that Acer and Bergalis had essentially the same virus. Myers recognized that the two shared some unusual combinations of bases, combinations not widely found in his data set. It was as if their faces shared a distinctive pigment in the eyes, a special contour of the lips, an unusual birthmark that revealed that they were indeed siblings. Myers, who had fully expected to show that there was no relationship between the viruses in Acer and Bergalis, was "astonished" at how "uncannily close" the sequences appeared.[26]

First impressions can be powerful, but they can ultimately mislead. Outsiders are certain to be skeptical of their merit. Myers did not know yet how to demonstrate that his insight regarding the unusual patterns was correct. As a result, he had to rely on somewhat more conventional, though imperfect, statistical analyses. These analyses involved two related techniques: genetic distance measurements and parsimony cluster analysis. The genetic distance between two cases of HIV is simply the proportion of nucleotide bases that differ between the DNA sequences. If 96 percent of the letters in two DNA sequences match up, for example, the genetic distance between them is 4 percent. The idea is that the greater the distance between the sequences of two persons, the less likely it is that one infected the other, while the smaller the distance, the greater the chance that the infections are related. Cluster analysis, in contrast, draws phylogenetic (essentially, family) trees showing how closely related each viral sequence is to the others. Sequences that cluster together to form branches are assumed to have a common ancestor, while those branches spaced farther apart are assumed to be only distant relatives. Genetic distance measurements and cluster parsimony analysis may be two different techniques, but they are not really two separate tests. As both techniques examine the same data, albeit in differing ways, they generally produce similar results, unless the sequences are only distantly related.

These techniques helped Myers determine the similarities in the viruses of Acer and Bergalis. Yet although the statistical techniques Myers used involve mathematical calculations, they do not produce a single correct answer regarding how similar the viruses are or whether they are similar enough to be related. In fact, the answers they produce are neither singular nor conclusive.

Measuring the similarity of the viruses depended entirely on how much of the viral DNA Myers examined and how he examined it, issues for which there was little clear guidance. (Due to technological limitations, he could not examine the entire virus.) As late as July 25, 1990—just two days before the *MMWR* announced the possible link between Acer and Bergalis—Myers was still changing the estimates he was providing Jaffe and Ciesielski. (The *MMWR* reported on July 27 that the sequences within Acer and Bergalis differed by an average of 4.5 percent; within Acer alone by 3.5 percent, and within Bergalis by 2.0 percent. On July 24 these figures were given more widely as 5.7 percent, 4.6 percent, and 2.3 percent, respectively.[27] The numbers continued to change because what Myers counted continued to change.[28] Perhaps this made the investigators at CDC headquarters a little nervous. To ease their minds, Myers wrote, "*No cause for alarm . . .* While [these changes] reduce the data set by about 20 percent, [they] greatly reduce the noise and lead to more defensible and cleaner comparisons."[29] Myers was not "stroking" the data to find what he wanted, but just "cleaning" it to help show what it contained.

Myers was not alone in being responsible for these initial calculations. Just as Leigh Brown had been called in to replicate Ou's work, James Mullins, a professor of microbiology and immunology at Stanford University, was brought in to recheck Myers's analysis. Mullins confirmed that Myers had taken the appropriate steps and made the sensible decisions.[30]

These estimates did not—and could not—provide a single definitive answer to the question of whether Acer infected Bergalis. The most that Myers's analysis could show, at the time of CDC's initial announcement, was that "the case reported here is *consistent* with transmission of HIV to a patient during an invasive dental procedure."[31] The summary of Myers's study in the *MMWR* was even more modest:

> The DNA sequence data indicate a high degree of similarity between the HIV strains infecting the patient and the dentist. . . . However, use of DNA sequencing for this purpose is new, and there is a paucity of sequence data pertaining to the HIV–1 viruses of sex partners and other epidemiologically related patients. The quantitative criteria for determining epidemiologic linkage based on HIV sequences are just now being developed.[32]

In contrast, by the end of Stage 2 the CDC reported there was little possibility (just 0.6 percent, or six in one thousand) that the DNA sequences from Bergalis, Webb, and Driskill "would be closer by chance alone to the sequence from the dentist than to the sequences from the eight local controls."[33] In other words, at that time the researchers indicated that they were 99.4 percent confident that it was no coincidence that Acer and these three patients shared the same cluster of viruses. This means that Myers and the others could be pretty certain that the dentist had infected these patients.

UNCERTAINTIES IN THE ANALYSIS

Yet although the quantitative criteria became more fully developed and the researchers grew more confident in them, the CDC still would never and could never say with certainty that Acer was the one. The reason for this is inherent in statistical analysis. The problem is basically this: just as two people might look alike either because they were actually related to each other or through pure dumb luck, two persons' HIV may look much alike either because they have a common source of infection or through random chance. What quantitative analysis does is set up procedures that allow the researcher to determine the probability that the viruses look alike due to luck or due to being related. Ultimately, the researcher is left only with these probabilities—often expressed in terms of the researcher's "confidence level"—that the relationship exists.

The story is actually more complicated even than this. The confidence level does not really mean that the researcher is, say, 99 percent confident that the conclusions from a particular test are correct. The confidence level indicates that if the test were performed an infinite number of times, it would provide the correct answer 99 percent of the time. Of course, the one test that the researcher performed might be the one yielding an incorrect conclusion.

Neither God nor nature dictates how high the confidence level must be for statisticians (and the rest of us) to conclude that relationships are real rather than random. Most often, statisticians do not conclude that relationships exist unless they have a confidence level of at least 90, or 95, or even 99 percent. But these confidence levels are arbitrary, as there is no particular reason that a researcher should conclude that a relationship does not exist if the confidence level is only 89, or 94, or 98 percent.

Moreover, the same confidence levels need not be used for every test. In general, the more important the issue, the higher the confidence one should have before concluding that similarities are real rather than random. Does the blood at the scene of a crime come from the defendant? If a guilty verdict means that the accused will be sentenced to death, justice requires that we be quite certain—that we have a high confidence level, since we want to be convinced beyond reasonable doubt—before answering yes. Still, opinions will vary as to how high this confidence level must be and how certain we must be. Those least in favor of the death penalty are likely to demand a much higher confidence level than those most willing to impose death on less convincing evidence.

It is easy to speculate, as many have, that CDC officials (or Myers) wanted to *prove that* (not *test whether*) Acer infected his patients. If Myers were able to show that the viral DNA of Acer and Bergalis were linked, for example, then he would be able to claim credit for having discovered the first case of doctor-to-patient infection—and uncovering such "firsts" is the road to scientific fame. Moreover, if the CDC were able to demonstrate that a physician transmitted HIV to patients, then the agency could demand greater authority and resources to prevent future transmissions. Indeed, the view that bureaucrats generate crises or exaggerate problems in order to gain power and resources is a common one in American political analysis.[34] Myers and the CDC both had selfish reasons, it would seem, to show that Acer transmitted HIV to Bergalis.

These speculations may seem plausible on the surface. In quantitative research, which Myers was doing, there is a clear bias toward finding "statistically significant" effects (that is, finding that relationships exist rather than showing that they do not). As one researcher put it, "investigators who find an effect get support, and investigators who do not find an effect don't get support. When times are tough it is extremely difficult for investigators to be objective."[35]

In addition, no fame awaited Myers on this project if he concluded that Acer and Bergalis had unrelated infections. (Myers, for his part, insists that fame did not motivate him and that he passed up numerous other opportunities to find it. Still, Myers did indeed obtain a measure of notoriety for his work on this project.) Thomas Edison, after all, became famous for inventing the electric lightbulb, not for finding hundreds of materials that didn't work. The CDC, for its part, was continually strapped for funds, especially in the 1980s and especially to conduct its research on the growing AIDS epidemic.

Why, then, would we not expect Myers and the CDC to juggle the data so that the results would lead to the conclusion that Acer infected Bergalis? A potential answer is that they also had selfish reasons to conclude that the infections were *not* related. For example, it is possible that the CDC would want most to maintain a cozy relationship with its medical constituencies as well as to calm the public, so it would want to deny that HIV is transmitted in medical settings.[36] One might also note that Myers has since spent much time testifying in lawsuits, meeting with skeptical interviewers, and fulfilling Freedom of Information Act requests—hardly glamorous or career-enhancing activities.

Still, if Myers and the CDC had self-interested reasons to find that Acer infected his patients—or to find that he did not—it is clear that they had stronger professional reasons to come to the correct conclusion, no matter what it was. In particular, competent scientific research calls for providing an explicit account of procedures and making data publicly available so that others may attempt to replicate results (as the CDC itself did during this investigation by having Leigh Brown double-check Ou's work and Mullins do the same for Myers). As it was obvious to the CDC that other researchers would be interested in scrutinizing the data—and at least a few persons would want to repudiate the official conclusions—they had a greater motivation to be correct than to be first. (Ultimately, the court of scientific opinion has supported the CDC's conclusions.[37]) Myers, for his part, responded with amazement when asked about any motivations he might have to manipulate the data. The data, he insisted, speak for themselves.[38]

They only speak, however, if they are helped to gain their voice. Accordingly, the researchers took measures to improve the validity, the accuracy, and the reliability of their tests as they moved from Stage 1 to Stage 5. For instance, Myers, Ciesielski, and others recognized early that they needed to improve the quality of their "control group"—those persons whose viruses would be compared with the HIV of Acer and his patients. Improving the quality of this group reduced the likelihood that Myers and Korber would find that Acer and his patients shared a common virus; an improved set of controls would also help convince others that the CDC's conclusions were the correct ones.

In Stage 1, the CDC did not choose controls with the most important features. In particular, none of the group was selected from the area near the dentist's practice. Instead, the group consisted of seventeen other "distinct North American isolates" for whom sequences currently existed at LANL.[39] Myers thus could not compare the genetic sequences of Acer and Bergalis to the sequences of similar individuals but only to other assorted individuals in the LANL registry. But if HIV had local population characteristics (so that two individuals from the same area would have quite similar strains of HIV even if they did not have a common source of infection), failure to include local individuals in the lineup could have biased the results to show incorrectly that Acer and Bergalis had related cases of HIV even if they did not. While Stage 1 was in progress, the possibility that HIV had local population characteristics had not been ruled out; on the other hand, there was also no strong evidence that such similarities did exist.[40]

The CDC's officials were well aware of this potential problem and started to remedy it even before the initial *MMWR* article on this case was released. Regarding Myers's Stage 1 analysis, a draft proposal to collect additional blood samples stated that "the results . . . *are inconclusive and can only be interpreted* if the isolates [of Acer and Bergalis] are compared with isolates from HIV-infected patients residing in the same geographic area to determine the prevalence of particular DNA sequences in the community" (emphasis added). A revised proposal removes this highlighted phrase and inserts instead that Myers's results "will be even more convincing."[41]

The CDC's Ciesielski attempted to remedy this deficiency in the following stages by collecting and analyzing blood samples from HIV-infected persons at two HIV clinics located within ninety miles of the dental practice. (These individuals were dubbed "local controls," or LC.) Ciesielski's team also obtained information on the patients' race or ethnicity, mode of exposure to HIV (male, sex with male; IV drug user; or other/unknown) and medical status (asymptomatic, symptomatic but not AIDS, and full-blown AIDS). No data were collected on the patients' length of infection or type of medical treatment, two factors that can influence how much variation exists in the genetic sequences. Severity of symptoms could serve as a proxy for the length of infection, however, as it typically took ten years after transmission for AIDS to develop.

In Stage 2, the CDC expanded its control group to include HIV sequences from eight LCs in addition to twenty-one sequences from the national HIV registry. Interestingly, one of the controls had been identified as a sexual partner and a patient of Acer's. This LC was "occasionally included in the analyses but not in the *MMWR* articles . . . [as] it is quite apparent that [his] sequences are not linked to the dentist's sequences nor to any of the other patients' viral sequences."[42] (Apparently, the CDC did not know what to make of this result and so simply omitted it.) In Stage 3, the CDC included an additional twenty-four LCs in its analysis. In Stage 4, a total of thirty-five HIV-positive individuals (including those selected in the earlier stages) were used in the comparison group; in Stage 5, five additional LCs were added to the data set.

How good was the comparison group? As good as was practical but not as good as could be desired: the researchers were pretty sure they were comparing apples to apples. Table 3.2 shows some of the characteristics that potentially affected HIV variation in the dentist, the patients, and the LCs at the time the CDC took their blood samples. (Less information is available concerning Patients H or J or Sherry Johnson; they are thus excluded from this table.) The table shows that these characteristics were neither identical nor randomly distributed across the patient and comparison groups, as they would be in the ideal scientific experiment. The LCs tended on average to have been infected for a longer period, to have a disease that had progressed further, and probably to have received more therapy than Acer's patients. Because the LCs differed systematically from the patients, it was more difficult to determine whether the differences in HIV among all these

Person	Duration of Infection, in Years [a]	Stage of Disease	Therapy	Apparent Source of Infection[a]
Dentist	More than 3	AIDS	AZT	Unknown
Patient				
A	Less than 2	AIDS	AZT	Dentist
B	Less than 2	Asymptomatic	None	Dentist
C	Less than 5	Asymptomatic	None	Dentist
D	Unknown[b]	AIDS	Unknown	Unknown
E	Less than 2	Asymptomatic	None	Dentist
F	Less than 2	Asymptomatic	None	Unknown
G	Less than 2	Asymptomatic	None	Dentist
H	Unknown[b]	Asymptomatic	None	Unknown
Local Controls	Unknown[b]	17 AIDS 10 Symptomatic 7 Asymptomatic	Unknown	Unknown

Table 3.2.   Factors Potentially Affecting HIV Variation: Status at Time of Blood Sample Collection
[a]As indicated by CDC's investigation.
[b]The average length of time between infection and diagnosis of AIDS is about ten years.
Source: U.S. Government Accounting Office, *AIDS: CDC's Investigation of HIV Transmissions by a Dentist* (Washington, D.C.: U.S. Government Printing Office, 1992), p. 27.

persons were attributable to the source of infection or to other reasons. Still, because Acer's characteristics with regard to HIV were more similar to the LCs' than to the patients', it might be expected that the dentist's strain of HIV would also differ from the patients if he were not the source of infection. Still, although the comparison group could have been even better, the steady progress in its quality shows that the CDC made good-faith efforts within the practical constraints (time, money, knowledge) to perform the soundest possible research.

CONFIRMING THE RESULTS

Good researchers can also use other methods to improve the reliability of their conclusions. One such technique is to increase the size of the sample, not by including more persons but by including more data—DNA sequences—from each person in the study. The rationale is that the more of the virus we examine, the better we are able to determine whether similarities are real or random. The best way to do this was to use multiple individual sequences (rather than "consensus" or directly amplified sequences) from the dentist, patients, and local controls. This, too, was done. By Stage 5, multiple individual sequences were used almost exclusively (except for some LCs).

Another way to improve reliability is to reduce the irrelevant information (or "noise") from the data. Myers did this, too, by focusing on the portions of the genetic material that could be clearly "scored" rather than the portions that were ambiguous or difficult to measure.[43] A third method to improve the trustworthiness of the results is to conduct multiple types of tests on different kinds of data. The idea is that if these different tests showed that Acer and his patient had related viruses we can have more confidence in this conclusion than if one only test showed this. To this end, Myers and Korber used genetic distance measurements, parsimony cluster analysis, and—as Korber told me—every other method of comparison they could think of.[44]

A final way to develop confidence in your conclusions is to create new and more accurate tests. Myers and Korber did that, too.[45] The genesis of the new test began with Myers's expert first impressions of the data. When Myers first examined the sequences of Acer and Bergalis, he noted that they shared a distinctive (and unusual) amino acid pattern sequence. (Amino acids are larger groupings of the nucleotide bases.) It was not just that the virus in Acer and Bergalis looked alike; it was as if they shared a common birthmark that no one else had. (Mullins, who reviewed Myers's analysis, noted that this unquantified visual evidence was "more compelling" during the initial stages of the investigation than the more formal existing statistical techniques showed.[46]) How, Korber and Myers wondered, could this observation be turned into a test that would objectively measure the uniqueness of this image?

They went about answering this question bit by bit. They reasoned first that a feature appeared unusual only when there was a "usual" to which it could be compared. They thus set out to discover what was the usual pattern of amino acids in HIV. Korber and Myers did this by lining up the amino acid sequences from a group of individuals having viruses in the HIV sequence databank and identifying the most common acid at each position. These most common acids became the "reference set." (Every individual did not have every amino acid in common with the reference set, but every position in the reference set had the most common amino acids among the individuals.) Next, these two scholars reckoned that Acer's virus would be considered unique at the points where all six of his sequences were different from those in the reference set. Korber and Myers found eight such sites, which became the dentist's "signature."

A comparison of Acer's signature and that of the reference group is shown in Table 3.3. Acer's signature consisted of the amino acids A, I, A, G, A, E, V, and H. Note that Acer had these acids at the same position in each of his viruses, while the reference set almost never did (at most, only 25 percent of the reference set had the same acid at the same position). Similarly, most people in the reference set had the amino acids E, T, E, S, T, A, I, Q at these positions, while this combination never appeared in Acer's virus. Like John Hancock's, Acer's signature was nothing like the others.

Korber and Myers then wondered whether Acer's signature would appear in the viruses of his patients, if he had infected them. To check this, they compared the amino acid sequences in the patients to Acer's signature and to the reference set. The results are striking. Acer's signature appeared almost exactly in Bergalis, Webb, Driskill, Shoemaker, and Yecs. (Bergalis and Shoemaker matched the signature pattern exactly on all of their sequences. Webb had an eight-for-eight match on eleven of her sequences and a seven-for-eight match on the twelfth. Driskill matched exactly on four of his sequences and matched seven for eight on the last. Yecs matched eight for eight on four sequences and seven for eight on two.[47]) Like Acer, these five patients had

Frequency in:	Reference Set's Amino Acid Signature							
	E	T	E	S	T	A	I	Q
1. Reference Set	63	81	69	59	69	66	72	56
2. Acer	0	0	0	0	0	0	0	0
3. Bergalis, Webb, Driskill, Yecs, Shoemaker	0	0	0	0	0	20	0	0
4. Patients D and F	55	100	73	91	0	45	82	82
5. Florida LCs	67	67	63	75	42	60	85	82

Frequency in:	Acer's Amino Acid Signature							
	A	I	A	G	A	E	V	H
8. Acer	100	100	100	100	100	100	100	100
9. Bergalis, Webb, Driskill, Yecs, Shoemaker	100	94	97	100	100	100	69	100
10. Patients D and F	36	0	0	9	100	0	0	0
11. Reference Set	6	13	6	16	25	6	25	16
12. Florida LCs	15	23	4	15	58	6	14	28

Table 3.3.   Signature Pattern Analysis (Frequencies in Percent)
Source: C.-Y. Ou, C. A. Ciesielski, G. Myers, C. Bandea, C.-C. Luo, B.T.M. Korber, J. I. Mullins, G. Schochetman, R. L. Berkelman, A. N. Economou, J. J. Witte, L. J. Furman, G. A. Satten, K. A. MacInnes, J. W. Curran, and H. W. Jaffe, Laboratory Investigation Group, Epidemiologic Investigation Group, "Molecular Epidemiology of HIV Transmission in a Dental Practice," Science 256 (May 22, 1992), p. 1168.

virtually nothing in common with the reference set at these positions. Patients D and F, however, appeared to have much more in common with the reference set than with Acer. Next, Korber and Myers compared the reference set and Acer's signature to the local controls. Once again, the LCs were much more similar to the reference set than to Acer. While the five patients matched Acer's signature almost perfectly, no LC was even close to an exact match.

Finally, Korber and Myers asked themselves how likely it would be for Acer's signature to appear in even a single sequence of Bergalis, Webb, Driskill, Shoemaker, and Yecs by chance (given how little this signature was found in the HIV-infected population as a whole). Using quite conservative assumptions (they used the single sequence of the patients that was least like Acer and the single sequence of the LCs that was most like him), Korber and Myers calculated that the probability that any single patient would have a pattern so much more similar than the LCs' to the dentist's by chance alone as 0.000008 (that is, eight in a million). This implies that the probability that Acer had two patients who matched him so closely by chance was roughly six in one hundred billion. There was virtually no chance that Acer could have six patients whose viruses so closely resembled his unless the cases were directly linked. This was the bull's-eye. In statistical terms, the signature pattern analysis came about as close to proof as it is possible to get that Acer, Bergalis, Webb, Driskill, Yecs, Shoemaker, and Johnson had a common source of HIV infection.

POSTSCRIPT

The field investigation had attempted to discover whether the patients contracted the virus outside the dental clinic; it was unable to do so. For each of the six infected patients, the only confirmed potential exposure to HIV came through Dr. Acer. The genetic analyses provided compelling, although not absolute, proof that Acer and at least six of his patients shared a very similar virus. Together, the field and genetic investigations produced overwhelming evidence that Acer had infected Kimberly Bergalis, Barbara Webb, Richard Driskill, Lisa Shoemaker, John Yecs, and Sherry Johnson.

The investigation was pathbreaking. For the first time, scientists concluded from blood samples—not behavior—that two (and more) persons had a common source of infection. The lessons from the research went far beyond this individual case. Korber and Myers, in trying to quantify and formalize Myers's first impressions about the "striking similarity" of the HIV in Acer and Bergalis, developed a new test ("signature pattern analysis"), and the computer program (VESPA) was created to conduct it. This test has since been widely used in AIDS research—for instance, to examine the matter of "superinfection," which is whether a person with HIV can be reinfected. If superinfection occurs, then each infection should have its own distinct signature pattern. If HIV does not have a fingerprint, it at least can have a distinct "signature."

In some ways this was science as usual. Scientific skills and knowledge typically improve over time as researchers form questions, gather data, conduct experiments, puzzle over the results of these experiments, and distribute their results for others to question. Scientific knowledge is tentative and subject to change. Definitive answers to important problems are difficult to find, especially when the problems are new and change over time. Because the CDC was breaking new ground and its study was exploratory, the researchers did not always have clear criteria to follow. The scientists were trying to develop the correct theories, the appropriate techniques, and the meaningful tests at the same time that they were trying to learn whether the fatal extractions had occurred.

Yet this case was also not just science as usual. The outcome of the research was of extraordinary interest to lawyers, the media, and the public. Myers, for his part, has stopped doing contract work for the CDC, despite his admiration for the agency. The turning point, he suggests, was the day he received a large stack of Freedom of Information Act (FOIA) requests for the data involved in this investigation. He wants to do research, he said, not comply with FOIA requests or testify in lawsuits.

The CDC's lab investigation provided convincing evidence that David Acer, Kimberly Bergalis, and at least five other patients of Acer shared a common strain of HIV, although this study did not show who infected whom. The field investigation by the CDC and HRS indicated that none of the patients had a documented exposure to HIV outside the dental clinic. Yet the question remained: How did Acer's patients contract HIV?

CHAPTER FOUR

Mystery
How Did Acer Do It?

C urran, Jaffe, Ciesielski, and other CDC and HRS officials knew that Acer was likely to have transmitted HIV to his patients in one of only three ways. He could have had sex with them. He might have operated on them with contaminated equipment. Or he may have directly exposed them to his blood. (Some have suggested that Acer might have infected his patients in some more novel way, such as by sneezing on them. While CDC officials no doubt pondered such possibilities, these were for all practical purposes impossible to investigate.) Yet within these simple possibilities were wrapped additional riddles. Did Acer have some sort of "supervirus" that made it easy for him to transmit HIV through tainted equipment? Did Acer infect each patient, or did the virus pass from patient to patient? Was Acer uniquely sloppy, and was this sloppiness induced by AIDS? Was Acer a sociopath who deliberately infected his patients by bleeding into their mouths?

The sexual transmission scenario was the easiest one to eliminate. All of the patients denied having sex with Acer. In addition, the patients told the CDC investigators—and Acer's dental staff confirmed—that Acer had never used a general anesthetic on them. It thus appeared most unlikely that he had sexually abused them while they were unconscious. The idea that Acer had infected his patients by having sex with them was rejected as quickly as it had been raised.

WAS IT CONTAMINATED EQUIPMENT?

A more intriguing—and potentially more ominous—possibility was that Acer's patients had become infected because he had treated them with contaminated dental equipment.[1] At least in theory, such transmission was clearly feasible. Dental tools, as any patient can attest, often become coated with blood during use. The tools' internal parts, unseen, can also be tainted. As HIV is carried in blood, it seems obvious that dental tools could then transmit the virus. But this surface truth must be subject to more critical and specific scrutiny. How easily do dental tools spread infection? What evidence is there that Dr. Acer's tools in particular were contaminated? Did Acer treat himself before operating on his patients? Or did tainted tools spread the infection from patient to patient? The answers to these questions are more difficult to come by.

When first asked how long HIV could remain infectious on dental equipment, Donald Marianos and Barbara Gooch, CDC dental surveillance officers, told me that it depends.[2] The ability of HIV to survive outside the human body is affected by several factors, such as the amount of blood exposed, the amount of HIV in the blood (called the virus's "titer"), and the temperature and humidity of the dental equipment's environment. The larger the pool of the virus, the higher the titer, and the more conducive the conditions, the longer HIV will remain infectious. So, Marianos and Gooch were asked, can HIV remain infectious on dental equipment? The frank answer in 1992 was this: We do not know. At the time that the CDC was trying to learn how Acer had infected his patients, there were simply no studies assessing the survivability of HIV on dental equipment (or any other kind of surgical equipment, for that matter).

There were a couple of worrisome signs, however. Since the early 1970s, at least thirty-three outbreaks of the hepatitis B virus (HBV) had occurred in medical clinics where the health care worker carried the virus, with more than 330 patients contracting the disease.[3] (It is interesting that these outbreaks did not create nearly as much public concern as the Acer case did, since many more patients have died from HBV than HIV contracted through medical care.) In these clusters of infections, as few as three or as many as fifty-five patients had contracted HBV. Nine of these outbreaks were linked to dentists. (All of the infections had occurred before 1987, however, prior to the time that public health officials began emphasizing more strongly that HCWs should be vaccinated against hepatitis and use universal precautions to prevent its spread.[4]) In addition, it had been demonstrated numerous times in laboratories that dental equipment could transmit bacteria.[5]

These findings were suggestive, but they were hardly conclusive, because the Acer case was not the only epidemiological mystery: no one knew exactly how the patients had been infected with HBV, either. In most cases, the physician was considered to be at a highly infectious stage of the disease. (The physicians who infected their patients were typically hepatitis B "e antigen," or Hbeag, positive. The presence of Hbeag is associated with higher levels of virus circulating in the blood and thus with higher infectiousness.[6]) Most of the infections also apparently occurred after the physician had performed a particularly "invasive" procedure (for example, dental extractions rather than cleanings). In each case, furthermore, there appeared to be a major break in infection control practices (for example, with the dentist not wearing gloves) or an injury to the physician. In no case could the infection be traced directly to a piece of dirty equipment, although in no case could tainted equipment be ruled out as a source of infection. And while lab tests had shown that bacteria could be spread through equipment, no study had proved that viruses—considerably more fragile—could be transmitted in the same way. As a result, the evidence from the HBV infections did little to tip the scales toward either the hypothesis of transmission through contaminated equipment or direct contact with the HCW's blood.

No dentist, we hope, would approach a patient with a visibly bloody dental tool. Even the most indifferent dentist would, we hope, at least wipe down the equipment with disinfectant between patients. The issue, then, was whether such a quick wipe-down would eliminate the virus (and hence the risk of infection) from the tool. As researchers began to examine this issue in detail, they soon learned that dental drills (typically called "handpieces")—already loathed by any sensibly pain-fearing patient—could harbor blood, saliva, and other material from the mouth of one patient and then spray it into the mouth of the next one.[7] How reassuring. Still, it was not at all clear that HIV could generally have a long life within a handpiece.[8]

Even more worrisome were a couple of recent surveys showing that the vast majority of dentists did not truly sterilize (by heating them in an autoclave) dental drills between patients; in one study, "more than 80 percent of [ten thousand dentist] respondents merely 'wipe' their handpieces for 'disinfection.'"[9] Still, despite this "extremely sorry state of affairs" regarding infection control in dental offices, it was nonetheless the case that no cases of HIV (or HBV, for that matter) infection had been documented from contaminated equipment.[10] This did not mean that such infections had not occurred. Because there were about 150,000 dentists and many millions of patients, a small number of infections from contaminated drills would have been easy to miss. (Remember, if Bergalis had not been adamant that she had no behavioral risk factors for HIV and if the investigation by Economou and Ciesielski had not confirmed this, it seems most unlikely that Acer would even have been suspected of spreading HIV to patients.) As the CDC's Jaffe summarized the issue early in 1992, while the CDC investigation was still very much alive, "it's quite clear that internal parts of these handpieces can be contaminated with blood. Whether it can result in the transmission of infection from one patient to another, we don't know. In theory, it could."[11]

It is one thing to suggest that contaminated dental tools can potentially transmit HIV; it is quite another thing to demonstrate that Acer's equipment actually did this. Indeed, it would be impossible to prove this—after all, there was no way to discover exactly what was on Acer's tools as they entered the mouth of Bergalis or the other patients. But it was conceivable that the CDC investigators could make a persuasive case based on circumstantial evidence that dirty equipment caused the infections. This case would have to be built on interviews with Acer and his dental staff, physical evidence from Acer's clinic, and reconstructing the timing and types of the patients' treatments. This is what we know about these matters.

David Acer opened his clinic across from a Toys-R-Us store on U.S. Highway 1 in Stuart, Florida, in 1980 when he was thirty-one years old. He had been working in a group practice in Opa-Locka, near Miami, before striking out on his own. He selected Stuart from among several locations, according to his mother, Harriett Acer, because "Stuart is very much like our hometown in North Canton [Ohio] where David grew up. It's a small, home-oriented town." To help build his business, Acer paid the local Welcome Wagon to distribute refrigerator magnets offering "a free teeth cleaning" on the first appointment with "Dr. David Acer—The Painless Dentist."[12]

Acer ran what seemed to be a typical dental practice. He employed an office manager (Maureen Englebart, who worked for Acer the entire time he was in solo practice), various dental hygienists, and other assistants. For a brief period between September 1985 and February 1986 he worked with an associate dentist, Elizabeth Greenhill. He and his staff performed all the regular dental services—cleanings, fillings, extractions, bridge placements, and crowns, for example. His patients came to him either through their own process of selection or through the recommendations or referrals of their insurers, especially CIGNA Dental Health of Florida. Turnover among staff was common, but no more common than in other dental clinics. When he became too ill with AIDS to continue practicing in June 1989, Acer sold his office to another dentist. After Acer closed the practice, he dispersed most patient records to other practitioners and threw out most of his office records (such as appointment books), keeping only the records of those patients who owed him money. His dental staff, with one exception, also left the clinic. Most of Acer's dental equipment was sold, and the office was remodeled.

The CDC had only one chance to talk with Acer about his infection control practices (when Ciesielski and Economou met with him at his home on March 29, 1990). In her summary of this meeting, Ciesielski briefly described Acer's account of his office's cleanliness: he did not heat-sterilize equipment after every patient but did use alcohol or some stronger disinfectant to wash the equipment.

This was not much to go on. To learn more about Acer's infection control practices, Robert Dumbaugh and Alan Lasch, Palm Beach County dental officers for the Florida HRS, identified, contacted, and interviewed all sixteen persons who had worked for Acer between 1987 and 1989. Both Dumbaugh and Lasch were themselves dentists. Dumbaugh or Lasch interviewed each staffer individually and later reinterviewed them all with CDC dental officers Marianos or Gooch. (The staffers were all tested for HIV, and none was infected.) A smaller group of the assistants were also questioned one final time on site at Acer's clinic.

In these interviews, Acer's staffers in general claimed to use appropriate infection control practices as a matter of routine.[13] For example, according to his staff, all surgical instruments were routinely heat-sterilized ("autoclaved") by 1987, while other heat-tolerant instruments were autoclaved as time allowed. Most other instruments were normally soaked in a disinfecting solution ("2 percent glutaraldehyde") between patients, "usually for at least twenty minutes."[14]

(Gooch notes that "HIV is unlikely to survive on instruments cleaned and then immersed in a 2 percent glutaraldehyde solution."[15]) Some equipment—such as prophylaxis angles, the "picks" hygienists use to clean teeth, and handpieces—was most often wiped with alcohol between patients. These interviews also suggested that by 1987, Acer, as well as his staff, wore latex gloves and surgical masks for patient care activities when appropriate. It seems that Acer and his assistants generally changed gloves between patients although, at least on occasion, the dental workers just washed their hands instead. Disposable anesthetic needles were used after 1983, and the staff reported no instances of needles that were reused on different patients. They did acknowledge that a single needle was routinely used multiple times on a single patient when multiple injections of local anesthetic were needed.

Still, it was difficult for Dumbaugh, Lasch, Marianos, or Gooch to verify the statements of the staffers or to determine how often breaches in infection control actually occurred. Acer's office had no written infection control protocols, no procedures for training staff in these protocols, and no policies for maintaining and documenting them. Although it appears that the infection control practices of the office improved over time, it is also pretty clear that Acer and his staff did not always follow "universal precautions" as specified in the CDC's 1987 recommendations or as Acer claimed in his open letter to the public. Acer's staff did not, for example, flush out handpieces after each use as the CDC recommended.[16]

The health officials had other reasons to be skeptical about the statements of Acer's staff regarding the sanitation practices used in his office. As the GAO reminds us, "statements of [the] dental staff should be viewed critically in the absence of supporting evidence. Because the dental staff had primary responsibility for maintaining infection control practices, disclosing breakdowns in these practices could put the staff in professional, financial, or legal peril."[17] The staff, then, had some reason to exaggerate how clean they kept the practice and to minimize any admission of sloppiness. Remember, also, that the CDC and HRS are public health, not law enforcement, agencies. Although the agencies' personnel sought to elicit the truth from the staffers, they had neither the power nor the predilection to compel the staff to tell it. Unlike law enforcement officers—who know that the subjects of their investigations are likely to lie—public health officials are normally inclined to accept the statements of other health care professionals as truthful.

Indeed, the legal testimony of these staffers provides a far less appetizing portrayal of Acer's practice. Elizabeth Greenhill, Acer's short-term associate in the mid 1980s, repeatedly urged him to improve his infection control practices. As she put it, "I was not 100 percent comfortable with his . . . office asepsis [sterilization techniques]."[18] Greenhill parted company with Acer over various differences in opinion about, among other things, patient care and practice routines. Still, Greenhill also testified that Acer's infection control "technique at that time was within the standard of care of the community."[19]

One dental hygienist, Margaret "Debbie" Crawford, worked with Acer during his final two years of practice. When Crawford was hired, "I explained to him that there were certain things I didn't feel comfortable with and that we needed to change them."[20] Crawford mentioned that the reuse of disposable saliva ejectors bothered her. She also reported seeing, to her dismay, that tools were placed in shallow disinfectant solutions that did not even fully cover the instruments and that blood splatters remained on the walls after Acer performed oral surgery. Crawford noted that even when instruments were sterilized in the autoclave, they were then dumped back into the tool trays rather than packed in sterile bags. As a hygienist, she demanded that Acer "clean up his office. It was filthy."[21] Diane Rubeck, one of Acer's assistants who began working for him about the same time, also stated that sterilization "wasn't done as a ritual. It would be done at their [the staffers'] convenience." Rubeck insists that she was fired because she was too vocal in her criticism of the office's infection control.[22] According to one account, Acer monitored his infection control in the following way:

> Dr. Acer would ask "How's our sterilization?" The staff would respond that everything was all right. The conversation would then turn to more important subjects, such as satisfying patients and increasing volume.[23]

Considered in isolation, these comments present a more damning portrait of Acer's dental practice. The problem is that from the broader perspective, Acer's clinic was not uniquely bad. As unpleasant as it sounds, Acer appears to have been not all that different from many other dentists regarding infection control.

So Acer was careless, at best, in the cleanliness of his office. The possibility that he infected his patients through tainted equipment may thus seem high. Yet if contaminated tools transmitted the virus to his patients, then the patients would have had to come into contact with these tools when they were infectious. There is no direct evidence that they did.

For the six patients to have contracted HIV by spreading the virus among themselves through tainted equipment, they would need to have had appointments one after another and have had the same dirty tools used on each of them. But these things did not happen. Although the dental records are very incomplete, the CDC's Gooch and Marianos were able to reconstruct, mainly from insurance records and patient interviews, appointment dates and types of treatment for five of the six patients.[24] (The sixth patient, Sherry Johnson, claims to have visited Acer several times during the summer of 1987, 1988, and 1989 for examinations, cleanings, and fillings. No information was available for treatment dates for Johnson, although an insurance record documents that Johnson was treated by Acer in August 1988, when her teeth were examined, X-rayed, and cleaned.) These records show that the patients tended not to visit Acer on the same days or to receive the same dental treatment when they did (Table 4.1). Kimberly Bergalis and Barbara Webb did visit Acer once on the same day (December 17, 1987), but Webb had a toothache (and so received an examination, X rays, and a prescription) while Bergalis had molars extracted under local anesthetic. Webb and Richard Driskill also both had their teeth cleaned on January 20, 1989, but neither received local anesthetic, nor was either patient given an "invasive" procedure. Acer's hygienist, Debbie Crawford, treated Webb; it is not clear who cleaned Driskill's teeth. Webb and John Yecs had two appointments in common. At the first, Webb received periodontal scaling—deep cleaning— and had an extraction, and Yecs was given a crown. It is not clear whether Yecs received a local anesthetic, although Webb most certainly did. Webb also had a bridge placement on August 29, 1988, the same day that Yecs had restorations on two molars. On this day both patients probably received a local anesthetic, but the other dental tools used on them would have differed.

Acer's infected patients thus received different treatments, on different days, over an extended time. The five patients made forty-eight documented visits to the dental office between November 1987 and June 1989. Webb had the highest number of documented appointments (twenty-one) and Shoemaker the fewest (two). On at least four occasions, two of the six infected patients visited the dentist on the

Date	Patient	Procedures Performed	Handpiece	Prophy. Angle	Anesthetic Syringe
December 17, 1987	Bergalis	Two molars extracted	No	No	Yes
	Webb	Exam	No	No	No
July 11, 1988	Webb	Tooth extracted; periodontal scaling	No	Yes	Yes
	Yecs	Crown replacement	Uncertain	No	No
August 29, 1988	Webb	Bridge placed	**Uncertain**	No	**Yes**
	Yecs	Anterior resin restoration	**Uncertain**	No	**Yes**
January 20, 1989	Webb	Cleaning	No	**Yes**	No
	Driskill	Cleaning	No	**Yes**	No

Table 4.1.   Procedures and Instruments for Acer's HIV-Infected Patients Who Shared Visit Days
ᵃBold type indicates dates on which the same instrument might have been used on both patients.
Source: B. Gooch, D. Marianos, C. Ciesielski, R. Dumbaugh, A. Lasch, H. Jaffe, W. Bond, S. Lockwood, and J. Cleveland, "Lack of Evidence for Patient-to-Patient Transmission of HIV in a Dental Practice," *Journal of the American Dental Association 124* (Jan. 1993), p. 40.

same day.[25] Could this just be a coincidence? Actually, it appears so. The probability of these occasions happening by chance alone is 60 percent; in other words, there is nothing unusual about this number of shared visits. (The CDC calculated this probability by assuming that patient visits occurred randomly on the days the dentist's office was open between the days of the first and last documented appointments of the patients and that no patient visited the dentist twice on a single day.) Furthermore, on only two of the four dates when two of the infected patients did visit Acer does it appear that the same dental tools *might* have been used on both patients. It just does not seem possible, given the available evidence, that the six patients infected each other through tainted dental equipment.

The possibility still remains that the equipment was infected by someone else and then used on these patients. But who? The most obvious suspect is Acer himself. Acer's hygienist Debbie Crawford indeed reported that she had cleaned Acer's teeth once and on one or two occasions had swabbed medicine on lesions on Acer's palate with a cotton-tipped applicator that she then discarded. Yet Crawford has also stated that she worked in a different treatment room than the ones Acer used, that she used her own instruments, and that she personally was responsible for their sterilization.[26] None of the staff members could remember Acer obtaining any other treatment at his own office, nor did they recall any episodes when he treated himself.[27] Acer did have an electrocautery that he used himself to burn the tumors on his palate, but as his assistants have confirmed, he kept this device at home and never used it on his patients.

The final possibility here is that some "mystery patient" contaminated the instruments. In this scenario, one of Acer's unidentified HIV-infected patients—a lover, perhaps—received treatment shortly before each of the six patients, the equipment was not cleaned between uses, and then the dirty tools were used to treat the Acer six. Like all conspiracy theories, this one contains a thread of plausibility. It is easy to believe that some dentists do, on occasion, provide treatment "off the books" to special individuals. Acer did, in fact, provide dental care to at least one person with whom he had had a sexual relationship. As we saw in Chapter Three, one of the local controls in the genetic sequencing study was identified as being both a sexual contact and a patient of Acer. It is inconvenient for this theory, however, that this person's HIV did not match Acer's or any of the other six patients.

Keep in mind, also, that most of the patients who were linked to Acer were able to claim large payments from Acer's insurer. As it would have been almost impossible to prove that the mystery patient had contracted HIV from sexual contact rather than from dental care, this person had a strong financial incentive to step forward. The failure of such a mystery patient to identify himself does not prove that the person does not exist. But the main support for the mystery patient theory, then, is that it has not been conclusively rejected. As such, we might as well name the mystery patient Elvis.

WAS IT ACCIDENTAL?

If the patients did not contract HIV through sexual contact with Acer or through contaminated dental instruments, then we are left with only one final possibility: they were infected through direct contact with Acer's blood.

The infections certainly could have happened this way. It has been well documented that HIV can be transmitted in health care settings; by 1990, approximately forty health care workers had already been identified who had been infected through occupational exposure.[28] It was also apparent that dentists do injure themselves at times while providing dental care. One survey of eighty-nine dentists revealed that almost one-third (32 percent) of them reported two or more "sharps" injuries per month; two of the dentists indicated that they injured themselves more than fifteen times each month.[29] (A "sharps" injury is one in which the dentist is cut severely enough by an instrument to draw blood.) A much larger survey (over 1,100 dentists) found that half of them suffered at least one sharps injury per month.[30] Dentists may also be more likely to injure themselves, it stands to reason, when they are tired, sick, or under unusual stress. And it is true that a substantial portion (between about 10 and 35 percent) of persons with AIDS suffer from "peripheral neuropathy," a temporary loss of control or trembling in the hands.[31] Since Acer had AIDS and thus suffered from illness, fatigue, and stress, and unless he was an exceptionally skilled dentist, he might easily have injured himself while caring for his patients.

Persons with full-blown AIDS, like Acer, are likely to have higher concentrations of HIV in their blood, which presumably makes them more infectious in general.[32] In addition, there is at least some evidence suggesting that some HIV-infected persons, for reasons still not fully understood, might be "supertransmitters." Epidemiologists have found that some people have infected virtually everyone with whom they have had intercourse; other individuals, in contrast, apparently are not very infectious, if at all. Some male HIV-positive hemophiliacs, for example, have had unprotected sex with spouses for long periods without infecting them.[33]

While this information shows that it was possible that Acer *could* have infected his patients through direct exposure of his blood, it hardly shows that he *did* infect them in this way. If anything, the medical literature at the time of the CDC's investigation suggested how improbable it was for HIV to be spread within health care settings. At the same time that the two surveys showed that dentists injured themselves fairly often, these same studies showed that no dentists had themselves been infected through their injuries. The forty-some HCWs who had contracted HIV through occupational exposure were only the tiniest fraction of that (unknown but large) number who had at some point come into contact with HIV-infected blood. At any rate, these studies provided only indirect data regarding the prospects for infection; firsthand evidence would have to come from Acer's dental practice.

Once again, what was most wanted was most lacking. Acer himself provided precious little information regarding injuries he might have suffered. Ciesielski's interview summary notes that "[Acer] does not recall any incident where he sustained a severe cut during a procedure. He does recall occasionally being stuck recapping the narrow gauge needle used to administer anesthetic, but said that usually the assistant would be the one stuck as she recapped the needle."[34] There is no direct evidence that he cut himself while treating Bergalis or any of the other infected patients.

But the CDC had two other potential sources of firsthand knowledge about Acer's dental practices—his staff and his patients. Yet neither could provide any evidence that Acer had injured himself while treating patients. At the time Acer was working, there was no office protocol for recording injuries (such as those suffered from needlesticks). In addition, none of the assistants could remember instances in which Acer had cut himself while providing treatment, even though the CDC and HRS investigators asked repeatedly about this. Nor could any of the infected patients remember a time when the dentist had wounded himself in a way that would have exposed them to his blood.[35]

Still, Acer was providing medical care while he was in the final stages of a terminal illness. He was diagnosed with AIDS in September 1987 when Kaposi's sarcoma developed on his palate, several months before he extracted Bergalis's molars. Acer started AZT therapy early in November of that year and received it almost continuously (except for a one-week period in December, when he experienced major side effects) until he closed down his practice in June 1989. For two weeks in June 1988, Acer was given radiation therapy for the cancer on his palate. According to his medical records and interviews with his health care providers, Acer suffered from fatigue but was relatively free of symptoms until March 1989. His medical records up to that point do not show any bleeding disorders, dermatitis on his hands, injuries, or dementia.[36] But the key phrase here must be "relatively free of symptoms"; while this may be accurate in comparison to other people with AIDS, a more important comparison would be to other practicing dentists. It has been reported, for example, that by January 1989 Acer had frequent coughing bouts

(Bergalis recalled this). An allergy to medication apparently caused him to have blurred vision and to miss over a week of work.[37] Yet by the time Acer's condition began to deteriorate rapidly, the infected patients had apparently pretty much finished their treatments.

The treatments that Acer provided each patient did create the potential for him to injure himself. All six of these patients received several injections of local anesthetic, and on each injection Acer conceivably could have stuck himself. Five patients (all except Johnson) were also treated in ways considered to be fairly "invasive." Bergalis, Webb, and Driskill had teeth pulled, for example, and Yecs and Shoemaker had root canals. Each of these patients was also given other treatments that certainly made him or her bleed and perhaps caused Acer to injure himself. Bergalis also had her teeth cleaned and had cosmetic bonding; Webb had periodontal scaling and obtained dentures; Driskill also had fillings, scaling, and bonding; and Yecs had fillings.

Sherry Johnson's case was the most puzzling. Unlike the others, Johnson neither had teeth pulled nor was she given a root canal. Her most aggressive treatment from Acer consisted of local anesthetic and restorative fillings.[38]

A summary is in order. The evidence is convincing that Acer did not infect his patients through sexual contact. It seems almost certain that he did not transmit HIV to them through contaminated equipment, although it is perhaps theoretically possible that he did so. It seems most likely that he infected the six patients by exposing them to his blood, yet there is no direct evidence from Acer, his staff, or his patients to confirm this. How, then, is it possible that Acer infected six people through exposing them to his blood? Only two hypotheses seem possible. The first is that Acer repeatedly cut himself and continued to work on the patients. The second is that Acer intended to murder his patients. Neither possibility is consoling. Neither hypothesis, moreover, has the kind of evidence that will convince skeptics. One of them, however, must almost certainly be correct.

There is nothing in Acer's record prior to his treatment of Bergalis in 1987 to indicate that he was too inept to practice dentistry. His dental school transcript shows that he graduated with a "B" average. His stint as a military dentist passed without problem, and he was honorably discharged. No complaints had been filed against him to the Florida dental board, nor had he been subject to any malpractice suits.

The fact that Acer was an average student, with no blemishes on his record and without malpractice suits, does not show that he was a competent dentist, however. One study found that only about one-half of 1 percent of physicians are sanctioned by disciplinary authorities each year and that only about 10 percent of these sanctions are imposed because the physician gave "substandard care." So while there are perhaps 150,000 to 300,000 victims of medical malpractice each year, only about 3,000 physicians—a tiny fraction of those practicing—are subjected to disciplinary action.[39]

Although any sign that Acer was incompetent prior to his treatment of Bergalis would provide evidence that he might have accidentally infected his patients, it is not true that this lack of evidence proves that Acer was proficient. Competence is not eternal; Acer could have been highly skilled earlier in his career, yet these skills could have deteriorated by the time he treated Bergalis and the others. Declining competence could have led to increasing accidents.

WAS IT MURDER?

It would have been easy, so it seems, for Acer deliberately to infect his patients. He had ready access to poison—his own blood—and he had compliant victims. It appears that it would have been a simple matter for Acer to draw some of his own blood and then inject it into the mouths of his patients as he was giving them local anesthetic. He needed only to escape the attention of his patients and staff while committing the murders.[40]

If this is what Acer did, then we should be thankful that he did not murder many more. No patient noticed anything suspicious in Acer's treatment—and none of the patients suspected Acer of murder. No staff member observed anything suspicious about Acer's patient care, and patients and staff members reported that Acer's staff assistants were typically present when he administered local anesthetic. If Acer had indeed injected his blood into his patients' mouths, this would have been no small deception, as he would have needed to break open a clear, single-use syringe of anesthetic, withdrawn some of it, and then refilled it with his blood, leaving the syringe visibly red. Acer then would have needed to administer this clearly tainted anesthetic in full view of patients and staff. Yet the fact that no one saw Acer use tainted syringes is meaningless to those who theorize that he murdered his patients; to the true believers, this lack of evidence *is* evidence of Acer's skillful malevolence.

One person who knew Acer has come forward to implicate his friend. Ed Parsons, a registered nurse from Miami Beach, claimed to have a five-year platonic relationship with Acer. During this time, Parsons claims, he grew to know Acer well as they played pool at Acer's home, went waterskiing, or hung out in bars. Parsons has argued that Acer was a heavy drinker who "resented society's opinion of AIDS and resented having to hide his homosexuality for fear of losing his practice."[41] Parsons quoted Acer as saying that "when AIDS finally infects a young person and when it starts hitting grandmothers and people like that, then maybe the government will do something." (This conversation allegedly took place at Roosters, one of the loneliest bars I have ever seen, in West Palm Beach.) Recalling one of their last conversations, in which Parsons claims he brought up the infections of Bergalis (the young person) and Webb (the grandmother), Parsons quotes Acer as responding, "I guess I've got their attention, don't I."[42]

The main weakness in this conversation is that it could not have happened. Bergalis was not publicly identified until after Acer's death, and Acer died before Webb had been diagnosed with HIV. There is no way that Parsons could have known that both these people had been infected while Acer was still alive. There are numerous other inconsistencies between the stories Parsons told to the press and those he gave while providing a legal deposition. Parsons, who was also HIV positive, contradicted himself regarding how he contracted the disease, whether his relationship with Acer was platonic, and his own sexual behavior, among other matters. Parsons was not a credible witness.[43]

Given that none of the potential witnesses actually saw Acer do anything devious and that the dentist made no confessions of guilt—in fact, he protested his innocence—there is precious little on which to convict him of murder. Yet the case can still be made, although it is a tricky one, that Acer's personality reveals that he was a serial murderer.[44]

In recent memory, the United States has had many highly publicized serial murderers—that is, a person who kills a succession of individuals, one at a time. Ted Bundy, John Wayne Gacey, Jeffrey Dahmer, among many other infamous brutes, first had their victims and then their biographers. Yet few serious efforts to develop psychological profiles of such men have been made. These studies have noted the great diversity among serial murderers, even while they have attempted to identify a few characteristics that they may have in common.

We must be clear, at the outset, as to what these profiles do and do not suggest. They do not imply that individuals with a certain type of family background, childhood experiences, or adult behaviors *will* or even *are likely* to become serial murderers. It should be freely acknowledged that the vast majority of persons with these characteristics will *not* become murderers. While the crime may reveal the personality, the personality does not cause the crime.

A more appropriate way to think about the relationship between psychological profiles and serial murders is to begin with the victims. The skilled criminologist will survey the bodies and ask, What sort of human could do this? The answer, it seems, is that only a certain distinctive individual could be capable of such cruelty; the crimes could only be committed by someone with a special personality. This means that if I only knew Acer himself, I would have no reason to suspect that he would murder six persons; yet because I do know that six of Acer's patients were slain, I might have cause from knowledge of Acer's personality to suspect that he did it. (As an illustration, the vast majority of "loners" are not serial killers, but almost all serial killers are loners. So if I learn that someone is accused of being a serial killer, then I will want to know if that person is a loner.)

The personal characteristics of serial murderers are varied and idiosyncratic: each murderer has been sick in his own way. But a long list of potential characteristics can be identified. But because this list is long and because no characteristics have been identified as essential, it is easy to show—depending on the ax you plan to sharpen—either that Acer was or was not like a serial murderer. Those who have judged him in print to be either sick or sane have never met him—nor have I—and so make their judgments based on second- or thirdhand information. With this in mind, let us look at the most compelling reasons to believe that Acer was innocent of murder.

Most serial murderers, it appears, are profoundly alienated from society, from their friends, careers, and especially their family. Acer was not. It is pretty clear that he was something of a loner, but it would have been hard not to be if you were gay and living in Stuart. And being a loner is not the same as being a drifter. He lived a conventional childhood, graduated on schedule from Ohio State University with a degree in predentistry, and then completed dental school (receiving his DDS at age twenty-six) in exchange for scholarship support from the Air Force Dental Corps. After serving his term in the armed forces, he was honorably discharged. He lived with his grandmother in Florida, establishing state residency, while he prepared for the state dental examination, which he passed on the first try. He worked in a group dental practice for a couple of years until he opened his own practice in 1980 when he was thirty-one years old.

His office manager, Maureen Englebart, worked and socialized with him the entire time that his practice was open, and she has vigorously defended him. His patients—even those who were infected by him— did not have mean words to describe him (although some considered him boring, and a few thought he was cold). On returning home after her first visit to Acer, Bergalis has been quoted as saying, "Dr. Acer seemed like a nice guy."[45] When asked under oath whether his office was clean, Kimberly's mother, Anna, replied, "Yeah, and the personnel [were] great. You know, it was kind of like a family type thing, really. . . . I mean, it was a professional, friendly atmosphere. . . . [Acer] was a pretty amicable guy."[46] As we have already seen, Acer described himself, in his open letter to the public, with these words: "I am a gentle man, and I would never intentionally expose anyone to this disease. I have cared for people all my life, and to infect anyone with this disease would be contrary to everything I have stood for."

Serial murderers, one might protest, are skilled at lying. If this was a lie, however, it was one bought by all those who knew him. His golf pro—and golf pros encounter liars as a professional hazard— remarked that Acer was "one of the nicest guys I ever met."[47] Linda Henry, who delivered Acer's magnets for the Welcome Wagon, called Acer her favorite sponsor.[48] Even Parsons, his accuser, has stated that Acer "was a very, very kind man, [a] very gentle man."[49]

Even more persuasive are his relations with his family. Acer was not estranged from his parents and siblings (even though, sadly, many gay men are). Throughout his life he remained on good terms with his mother, stepfather (his biological father died at the age of thirty-nine, and his mother remarried), his sister, and two brothers. In May 1989, when his health was deteriorating, he asked his mother to come to Florida to be with him. By June, both of his parents had moved to Acer's home to care for him, and Acer had willed his home to his mother. Whenever Acer was admitted to a VA hospital in Miami, his parents checked into a hotel nearby. Mildred Gelfand, a social worker who on several occasions counseled Acer after he was diagnosed with AIDS, wrote this in her patient records in August 1989:

Met with [Acer] and parents in the clinic and on the ward. This is a close-knit, loving family who are attempting to cope with [Acer's] illness. Following the transfusion, [Acer's] color returned. . . . This was a hopeful sign to his parents, who take a positive and spiritual approach to the virus. They received much consolation from a book sent to them by [another] son called *How Will I Tell Mother,* which discussed the issue of how to inform parents that their son's homosexuality was responsible for contracting the AIDS virus.[50]

In the summer before his death, Acer regained enough strength to travel with his parents to visit his brothers, sisters, and others in Ohio and Pennsylvania one last time. He then returned to Florida, where his parents stayed with him until he died. After his death, Acer's younger brother, Kenneth, said, "David was a kind, private man who meant harm to no one. I loved the man."[51]

If most serial murderers take no pleasure from their families, they do from killing. Acer could not have had such gratification. If he were a murderer, it must be the only case in history where the perpetrator died before his victims. And while most serial murderers apparently are obsessed with a particular type of victim—Bundy favored young women and Gacey and Dahmer had a taste for young men—Acer's patients were an eclectic group in gender and age: they included a girl, Johnson, who was a teenager when she was infected; a young woman, Bergalis; an adult woman, Shoemaker; a matron, Webb; and two adult men, Driskill and Yecs. This would constitute an exceptionally wide-ranging fetish. It is hard to see any feature that these individuals had in common other than that they all needed dental treatment.

It has been suggested that Acer was different from the "typical" serial murderer in that his patients were the victims of political terrorism. (In a political assassination, the perpetrator has a particular individual, such as the head of state, as a target. A political terrorist, on the other hand, is more interested in killing a particular class of individuals and not especially concerned if others die in the cross fire.[52]) This is implicitly the case that Parson made when he suggested that Acer wanted to target "valued" persons (in other words, those other than gay males) for whom the government would rush to find a cure for AIDS. On the surface, this argument might seem more plausible than the one concerning serial murder. It is true that the federal government was slow in addressing the AIDS epidemic.[53] The federal government's lethargy in finding a cure for AIDS and its reluctance to spend money for prevention or treatment during the early years of the epidemic are no doubt due in part to the fact that AIDS has hit hardest those for whom "mainstream" society has least sympathy: gay males, IV drug users, and ethnic minorities. It would certainly be understandable if Acer, infected with a fatal virus, had been angry at the government and interested in shocking it into taking action. Anger, after all, is one step toward confronting death.[54] And a central message of some AIDS organizations, like ACT-UP, is that the government *must* be shocked into action.

If Acer was a terrorist, he was an odd one. His targets, who could have been deliberately chosen, would hardly have been expected to alarm the government. Driskill and Yecs already resembled the typical person with AIDS: white, male, in their thirties, sexually promiscuous (although they were not gay), drinkers, and drug users. It is hard to imagine that Acer would infect these men to make a political point. Yet even Bergalis, Johnson, and Webb were hardly unique. Already by 1987 there were 365 girls and young women (below age twenty-four) diagnosed with AIDS; two more, Bergalis and Johnson, would not have caused the public to notice. In addition, at that time 175 women over the age of sixty had come down with AIDS. One must have a vivid imagination to think that Webb's case would have made governmental officials or the public sit up and say, "We'd better do something about this AIDS thing."

Political terrorists are under no obligation to be reasonable in their beliefs and sensible in choosing their targets, of course. Terrorists routinely kill individuals whose fatal mistake was to be near the terrorist. The link between the terrorists' victims and the terrorists' purposes is often obscure. In these respects, Acer might be no different from other terrorists. But in other ways, AIDS had hardly transformed Acer from gentle man to zealot. He had not pledged allegiance to any extremist organization. He had not joined any crusade. He had not devoted his life to any cause. As far as we can tell, Acer continued to lead a private life until his death. If he were a terrorist, he would be a curious one, although he would not have been *uniquely* solitary. The terrorist known as the "Unabomber," who specialized in sending mail bombs, had killed at least three people and injured more than a dozen between the late 1970s and 1995. Although the Unabomber's targets might appear to be chosen almost at random, it does at least seem clear that the perpetrator had an explicit political agenda. Acer had none.

The quality of the CDC's investigation of the murder hypothesis was weak—if we look at the CDC as though it were a police department.

But its officials are not law enforcement officers, and there are good reasons why the CDC did not pursue the homicide theory more vigorously. These reasons are based both on the way the case unfolded and on the CDC's role and responsibilities as a public health agency.

It would have been a different matter if all six victims had been identified at the same time: perhaps then the CDC investigators would have been more inclined to suspect foul play. In the opinion of many, including CDC officials, the prospects that Acer committed murder grow larger the greater the number of patients found to be infected by him. With each additional infection, the probability that they could all have happened by accident accordingly shrinks. But only one patient, Kimberly Bergalis, was linked to Acer before his death, and until just months before he died, the CDC considered it unlikely that Acer was the source of the infection. This meant that the CDC had only a short time to question Acer before he died, but this did not seem to be a problem because the CDC had little reason to suspect him of murder.

Remember, too, that Acer cooperated with Ciesielski and Economou when they first interviewed him (providing them his blood sample, a most incriminating piece of evidence); his lawyer then advised him not to participate in additional interviews. The CDC could not compel Acer to talk further, as it does not have the power to issue subpoenas. Nor could the CDC subpoena others who might have been able to shed more light on Acer's personality and his practice. Law enforcement agencies could issue such subpoenas, but they saw no reason to. Jaffe has noted that Florida's state's attorney office consistently stated that there simply was not enough evidence of murder for it to proceed with an investigation.[55] (Granted, from a legal perspective, there was no point to move forward with an investigation. The would-be defendant was already dead.) Even now, the best evidence that Acer intended to infect his patients is that the infections are difficult to explain in any other way.

MY VERDICT

This chapter ends with a puzzle. We can be almost certain that Acer infected at least some of the six patients. Yet if we examine the possible ways that he could have infected the patients—through sexual contact, contaminated equipment, accidental exposure, or deliberate malice—we find substantial evidence against every one of them. But surely the infections *must* have occurred in one of these ways. This is why the term "great mystery" will not go away. Despite the best efforts of the CDC officials—and numerous other individuals who have considered the evidence—we simply do not know how Acer infected Bergalis and the other patients.

Like those who ponder the full range of evidence rather than those who select the data that support their preconceptions, my own view shifts from day to day. When I consider that a single dentist transmitted HIV to six patients and that no other physician has been implicated in infecting even one patient, it is tempting to conclude that Acer must have done it deliberately. That the most invasive procedure performed on Sherry Johnson involved injecting a local anesthetic reinforces the view that the infections were intentional. But in reflecting on what I have learned about David Acer as a person—and virtually all of this evidence is thirdhand—it is difficult for me to believe that he murdered these patients. It is hard for me to picture Acer fooling his patients, staff, and, most of all, his family. It simply does not feel right.

Forced to decide whether the infections were accidental or intentional, we might hold an imaginary trial in which Acer was accused of six counts of murder in the first degree. If Acer is convicted, he would receive the death sentence. Given the evidence that has been presented, would I vote to convict? Is Acer guilty beyond reasonable doubt of murder? On these questions, my vote must be "No," although I acknowledge that some have been convicted on less evidence—and others have been acquitted on much more. This vote means "not guilty," of course, rather than "proved innocent." This, to say the least, is not an entirely comfortable conclusion.

The CDC officials, for their part, are no more comfortable. Although it used more than two dozen investigators and spent more than $1 million on its inquiry, the CDC remains officially uncertain about how the infections occurred. Harold Jaffe has spoken frequently about the CDC's disappointment regarding its inability to determine how Acer infected his patients.[56] When asked directly about which theory he believes to be true, Jaffe candidly responds,

I haven't a clue. There is no direct evidence for any of [the] theories. . . . Whatever happened with Acer has to be very unlikely because as far as we know it never happened before and as far as we know it has never happened since. With Acer, all the possibilities we are picking over seem to be wrong, and yet, one has to be right.[57]

The frustration from not solving the case deepens with time. All the data say something strange happened in that dental practice, and I wish I knew what it was. The fact that there were so many infected patients and there is no other practice like this may give more weight to the murder theory, but there is no proof of that. The only way it will ever be solved is if the dentist told somebody what happened, or someone saw what happened, and that person ultimately comes forward.

Obviously, we'd really like to know what happened, but at this point I'd be surprised if we ever get an answer. . . . Maybe, if Sherlock Holmes were a CDC employee, I could tell you what happened.[58]

Ultimately, little about this case was elementary. Anyone who suggests otherwise has not fully considered all the evidence. We conclude this chapter still asking how Acer did it.

CHAPTER FIVE

Conflicts

Patients vs. Experts

———✺———

Once the CDC announced that a dentist in Florida had possibly transmitted HIV to a patient, the media swarmed West Palm Beach to identify the mysterious "Patient A." Knowing that reporters would soon find them, the Bergalis family (on the advice of their attorney, Robert Montgomery) held a press conference on September 7, 1990. Before a room packed with all the major media, Bergalis told the world that she was the individual infected by the dentist. Montgomery also announced that the Bergalises had filed suit against Acer's estate.

But the press conference also had a larger purpose. Montgomery, while introducing the family, emphasized that the Bergalis family was not just seeking to collect damages; they also wanted to change public policies regarding AIDS in the health care workplace. Bergalis's father pleaded that "no one should have their daughter's life taken away. [Kimberly's] only shortcoming was her faith in the health care agencies. They failed and she paid the price. The guidelines in this country need to be changed. The rights of both health care workers *and* patients must be protected."[1]

Later, in a highly publicized letter released shortly before her death, Bergalis wrote:

> Who do I blame? . . . I blame Dr. Acer and every single one of you bastards. Anyone who *knew* Dr. Acer was infected and had full-blown AIDS and stood by not doing a damn thing about it. You are all just as guilty as he was. You've ruined my life and my family's. . . . P.S. If laws are not formed to provide protection, then my suffering and death were in vain.[2]

But what exactly should these laws be? The Bergalises had clear opinions, and so did many others. The problem was that these opinions were just as clear in their differences. Patients and experts had strong views and strong disagreements about what should be done to prevent transmission of HIV in the medical setting.

PATIENTS WANT PROTECTION

Let us consider first the issue through the eyes of a single patient, Kimberly Bergalis. She believed she had avoided exposing herself to HIV by refraining from risky sex or drug use. How might she have lowered her risks of contracting HIV from Dr. Acer or any other health care worker? She could, of course, have refused all medical care—an option that poses its own, potentially catastrophic risks to health.

A second option would have been for her medical providers to refrain from providing medical care if they were infected. Bergalis's father forcefully advocated this approach, arguing that "someone who has AIDS and continues to practice is nothing better than a murderer."[3] Alternately, her provider might have told her that he was HIV positive before treating her, thus giving her the option of accepting or rejecting his care. This is what Bergalis sought: "I'm not asking that we . . . live in a risk-free world. I want people to be able to choose their risks. I didn't have a choice to walk out of the office and seek another dentist."[4]

The Bergalises had reason to be skeptical that HIV-infected HCWs would voluntarily either tell this to their patients or stop practicing: Acer, certainly, had done neither. The clear implication was that for patients to be safer, the government needed to require HCWs infected with HIV to disclose or withdraw.

But how would the health care workers know if they are infected? A patient might expect them, out of concern for those they treat as well as for their own health, to get tested voluntarily. (Acer had done this.) But a patient might also worry that large numbers of HCWs might not get tested out of fear, denial, malice, or laziness. Patients might therefore demand that HCWs be required to be tested routinely. Without regular, mandatory tests to establish whether HCWs were infected, requirements for patient notification or practice restrictions would be hollow.

Sanford Kuvin, a medical consultant to the Bergalis family, strongly advocated that the government require HCWs to submit to HIV tests. Only in this way, Kuvin argued, could patients be protected and additional infections prevented. Mandatory testing, moreover, would not be a revolutionary innovation. Such testing has long been a staple of public health policy, as certain categories of diseases and particular groups of individuals have often—although not without controversy—been subjected to tests. Pregnant women face mandatory testing for syphilis and the hepatitis B virus, for example, while by the late 1980s those joining the military or the foreign service were required to undergo testing for HIV.

In the eyes of the Bergalis family, then, sensible public policies would contain compulsory routine testing of HCWs for HIV, and those testing positive would be automatically excluded from treating patients or, alternately, compelled to announce the test results to them. The central elements of the Bergalis position were that patients wanted and needed these protections and that the government ought to provide them.

The public—that is, the broadest group of patients—appeared to agree. Even before the Bergalis case, an overwhelming majority (80 percent) of the respondents in a national poll said that HCWs should be screened for HIV.[5] Almost a year after Bergalis's press conference, a substantial portion of the public agreed that HIV-positive HCWs must be forbidden to practice, with 65 percent thinking that HIV-positive surgeons should be barred, 60 percent holding that view about dentists, 51 percent agreeing that all HIV-positive physicians must discontinue practicing, and 49 percent believing that *all* HIV-positive HCWs must stop providing patient care if they are infected.

Support for patient notification was almost unanimous. A Gallup poll of a nationally representative sample of adults showed that about

90 percent of the public believed that all HIV-positive HCWs must disclose this fact to their patients, and 95 percent of the public believed that HIV-positive surgeons must notify patients of their HIV status.[6] The public, like the Bergalis family, thus wanted HCWs to be tested for HIV and compelled to disclose the results to their patients or stop caring for them—and the public wanted the government to respond to these desires.

EXPERTS PREFER DISCRETION

The majority of experts in health policy have rejected most of the Bergalises' policy ideas. Being experts, they have written about these issues at great length, in great detail, and with great sophistication. (Appendix Two lists some of the important articles. The articles by Larry Gostin and Mark Barnes are especially instructive.) I encourage you to examine these texts, as only a few highlights are presented here.

Testing

The call for mandatory testing has received the strongest opposition, for both practical and philosophical reasons.[7] On the practical side, mandatory testing of HCWs was seen as a very costly way to save lives. The ratio of costs to benefits was impossible to estimate precisely, however, as it depended on variables and unknowables. The costs depended mainly on the price of the test, the number of HCWs tested, and the frequency of the tests, along with the administrative costs of keeping records, counseling those who tested positive, and protecting their confidentiality, among others. A final hard-to-estimate cost involved the loss of medical expertise caused by removing those who test positive for HIV from providing medical care.

The benefits depended mainly on the unknown—and unknowable—number of patients whose lives would be saved because they would not be infected by HIV-positive HCWs. Because the costs and benefits could only be estimated, and the estimates depended on assumptions, the expected value of testing varied dramatically. One study suggested that mandatory testing would cost between $1 million and $90 million for each infection averted (other studies have given even higher costs)—an expense "much greater than that of other interventions determined to be a reasonable use of our health care resources."[8]

Still, it is worth noting that there is extraordinary variation in the cost effectiveness of different regulations, with some saving both money and lives and others costing many millions to save a single life. One analyst has identified more than a dozen regulations that appeared to cost more than $1 million (in 1985 dollars) per life saved, with the most expensive rule costing over $100 million per life.[9]

Another strike against mandatory testing came from the practical difficulties of administering the tests. Consider the example of a single dentist. Each working day the dentist is exposed to the blood of patients who might themselves be infected with HIV. The dentist might be tested for HIV today and prove not to be infected—but what about tomorrow, after additional dentistry is performed? Because many HCWs are exposed daily to patients' blood, the results of the HIV tests for HCWs would essentially be obsolete the day they are given. Frequent testing would still identify, fairly quickly, the HIV-positive HCWs, but it would simply not be possible to identify all infected HCWs the moment they are infected.

Civil libertarians also opposed mandatory testing for ethical reasons. Two were most important. Mandatory testing used the coercive power of government in a most intrusive way. In essence, the government would "search" individuals who were not suspected of wrongdoing and "seize" blood from them. Yet the Fourth Amendment to our Constitution explicitly guarantees the right of individuals to be free from unreasonable searches and seizures.[10] In addition, the test provided no particular benefit to those tested, since in 1991 there were no particularly effective treatments for HIV. (This is now changing as more effective medicine is developed.) Instead, those who tested positive faced personal, social, and economic hardships as a result. HIV was not, despite the wishes of some, just another disease; testing positive for HIV is not like testing positive for, say, hepatitis. Contracting HIV was seen as fatal and disgraceful, while contracting hepatitis was generally neither.

These points are illustrated by Acer himself. When he suspected that he had developed AIDS, Acer traveled a couple of hours south to be tested and to seek medical care in Fort Lauderdale; there, he used an assumed name (David Johnson). He never let his staff or patients know that he had AIDS, insisting instead that he suffered from cancer. Although some might see this as a sign of Acer's devious nature, a better interpretation is that Acer correctly believed that his community and his patients would shun him if they knew he were HIV positive.

There is a final, unsettling objection to mandatory testing for HCWs. Bergalis strongly argued for giving patients the choice to accept or refuse medical care. Why should HCWs have any less choice regarding the care—including testing—with which they are faced? If patients are to be given this choice, then it seems that the HCW, in this role also as patient, should have the same ability to refuse unwanted care.[11]

Mandatory testing was not totally unacceptable to civil libertarians, but they insisted that there be a compelling public benefit if testing were to be instituted. After the initial misgivings, there was little opposition to the idea that blood donors should be tested, for example. It was clear that the blood donation created an imminent threat to the recipients, while the test created little direct harm to the donor, so long as the results were kept confidential. It was not at all obvious that there was a clear public benefit to testing HCWs, however, particularly because not a single case (including Bergalis's) of *accidental* infection of a patient by an HCW had been demonstrated. To prevent deliberate infections, we would need a test for evil, not HIV. Still, many experts were sympathetic to the idea that HCWs, like all others, should voluntarily submit to testing if they thought they had been exposed to HIV.[12]

Even the most expensive and elaborate testing programs would not work perfectly, then, but would only reduce the possibility that HIV-positive HCWs would be unaware of their condition. This meant that testing was not "the" answer to the problem of HIV in the medical workplace but only one answer among many, with each having various costs, benefits, weaknesses, perversities, and uncertainties. Those who opposed mandatory testing thus were not necessarily preoccupied only with protecting the rights of those infected with HIV; they had also concluded that such testing was not the most appropriate answer to a public health problem.

Practice Restrictions

Let us put the testing question aside for a moment and address what might, at the outset, seem to be a simpler issue: should the practice of an HCW known to be infected with HIV be restricted? Part of the answer does seem easy. Most HCWs perform jobs that pose no risk (except a hypothetical one) of exposing their blood to their patients. (It is possible to conjure up some risk from every infected HCW— and from everyone else for that matter. Still, the idea that an HIV-positive orderly whose sole job is to change bedsheets might pose a risk to patients because the orderly could become scratched on a bedpost is, to say the least, imaginative.) The experts conclude that those HCWs who do not perform any "seriously invasive" procedures pose zero threat of infecting patients and therefore should not have their jobs restricted. (Even so, Gostin noted in 1990 that the HIV-positive HCWs who most often encountered practice restrictions were those who pose no risk to patients.[13])

A more perplexing issue involved those HCWs who performed "seriously invasive" procedures, the procedures with the greatest potential for infection. Here the case might seem the strongest for restricting HIV-positive medical providers. But even this case was not ironclad. Prevailing codes allowed HCWs infected with the hepatitis B virus (HBV, another serious and potentially fatal disease) to continue doing these procedures until it became documented that they had infected a patient. Some questioned why HIV-positive HCWs should have their practices automatically restricted given that HBV-positive HCWs did not.[14]

Restricting the practices of HIV-positive HCWs might, furthermore, illegally discriminate against their rights as "disabled" individuals. To understand this definition and these rights, we must step back for a moment from the particulars of this case to examine the evolution of disability policy.

Historically, people with physical or mental disabilities have faced serious discrimination in the workplace. Employers were reluctant to hire and anxious to fire workers who were disabled. To counteract this discrimination, in 1973 Congress enacted the Rehabilitation Act, the first major federal law to define and protect the rights of those suffering from physical impediments. Based in part on the Civil Rights Act of 1964, which protected racial minorities from employment discrimination by private employers, the Rehabilitation Act stated that:

No otherwise qualified individual with a disability in the United States . . . shall, *solely* by reason of her or his disability, be excluded from the participation in, be denied the benefits of, or be subjected to discrimination under any program or activity receiving Federal financial assistance.[15]

In their defense, employers could argue that the disability would harm job performance. Accordingly, employers were often unwilling to hire such persons not *solely* because of the disability but because they viewed the disability as reducing the employee's effectiveness. To resolve the conflict between employees who claimed that their performance was not hindered by a disability and employers who claimed it was, the federal courts adopted the following standard: the act prevails if the disabled employee "can perform the essential functions of the position in question without endangering the health and safety of the individuals or others."[16]

The boundaries of the Rehabilitation Act (regarding what it meant to "endanger health and safety") were further clarified in 1987 in the Supreme Court's ruling in *School Board of Nassau County* v. *Arline.*[17] Gene Arline had been hospitalized with tuberculosis in 1957, but then the disease went into remission for nearly twenty years. Ms. Arline began teaching elementary school in Nassau County in 1966. In 1977, however, her tuberculosis became active again. After her third relapse, in November 1978, the school board suspended her without pay for the remainder of the school year. At the end of that year, the board fired her "not because she had done anything wrong" but because of the "continued reoccurrence of tuberculosis."[18] Arline sued the board because she was fired solely because of her illness, which was, in her view, a disability.

The Supreme Court, by a vote of seven to two, agreed: a disease— even a contagious one—could be a disability under the terms of the Rehabilitation Act. In particular, the Court ruled that diseased individuals "could not be denied jobs because of the prejudice or ignorance of others. The Act replaces such fearful, reflexive reactions with actions based on reasoned and medically sound judgments as to whether contagious handicapped persons are 'otherwise qualified' to do the job."[19]

The Court held, moreover, that employers could not, in most cases, make blanket decisions excluding persons with certain disabilities from certain jobs. Instead, "individualized inquiries" should usually be made as to whether the disabled person is able to do the job, and "reasonable accommodations" must be provided for that person's special needs. A person with a contagious disease was "otherwise qualified" unless "reasonable medical judgments" determined that the person created a *"significant"* health and safety risk due to

1. The *nature* of the risk (for example, how the disease is transmitted)
2. The *duration* of the risk (how long the carrier is infectious)
3. The *severity* of the risk (what is the potential harm to third parties)
4. The *probabilities* the disease will be transmitted and will cause varying degrees of harm[20]

The American Medical Association, in an amicus brief submitted to the Court, had suggested these four criteria.

In this decision the Court explicitly refused to consider whether all persons infected with HIV were disabled.[21] In 1988, however, the Department of Justice announced that all people with HIV were protected by the act.[22]

The Americans with Disabilities Act (ADA), enacted shortly before the Bergalis case was announced in 1991, and its implementation by the Equal Employment Opportunity Commission (EEOC) further elaborated policies for the impaired.[23] Several extensions are especially noteworthy. Individualized evaluations, rather than blanket exclusions, became the rule, unless the impairment prevented the employee from conducting an "essential function" of the job. As driving a car is an essential function of a chauffeur's job, for example, it is not discriminatory to exclude all blind persons from becoming chauffeurs. It would be discriminatory to exclude all amputees, however, if a particular one had the skill to drive a properly equipped car.

On the issue of what constituted a "significant" health and safety risk, "an elevated risk of harm does not suffice; the risk must represent a high probability of substantial harm."[24] A reasonable accommodation is "any change in the work environment or in the customary manner of performing essential job functions that enables an individual with a disability to attain an equal level of performance . . . as the average similarly situated employee without a disability."[25]

Disability law thus had several implications for those who wanted to restrict HIV-positive HCWs. Most clearly, it had to be recognized that these HCWs were disabled and thus protected by the law; policies had to take this into account. In addition, HIV-infected HCWs could not be excluded as a group from providing health care unless this disability prevented HCWs from performing essential job functions. This would be the case, however, only if the HCWs were highly likely to cause substantial harm. Even then, if the HCW's work environment could be changed in such a way as to allow performance equal to that of the ordinary health care worker, the infected HCW could not be barred from practicing.

Still, the implications of disability law only begged the questions. Did HIV infection prevent certain HCWs from performing essential functions of their jobs? Were HIV-infected HCWs *highly* likely to cause substantial harm? And could their work environments be altered so that they could perform as well as their average uninfected peer? Even if the legal principles were clear, the factual answers to these questions were open to dispute.

Patient Notification

A final, even more difficult question concerned the responsibility of an HIV-positive HCW to reveal this fact to patients before treating them. The experts tended to conclude that HCWs, even those who conducted the most invasive procedures, did not have an obligation to reveal their HIV status to patients. This tendency was not absolute, as strong divisions existed within the medical community.

The idea of "informed consent" is often given as the rationale for patient notification. Patients, in this view, cannot make an informed decision to accept treatment unless they know the HCWs' HIV status. But there are a couple of weaknesses to this interpretation. Historically, the principle of informed consent was developed to assist patients as they made decisions regarding particular *treatments* (not physicians) with the view that patients could better make these decisions if they knew about the treatments' most important potential consequences. Rare risks need not be revealed, however. Informed consent, as a legal principle, has not required HCWs to provide information about their competence in providing the treatment. It was left to the licensing boards to ensure that each HCW was competent to conduct the treatment.

There are good reasons why HCWs give information about the risks of various treatments to patients without discussing their competency in delivering the treatments. Regarding treatments, both HCW and patient have an interest in seeing that the appropriate treatment (given risks and benefits) is provided. But the HCW and the patient do not have matching interests regarding the HCW's ability to provide the treatment. Here, the patient will want only the most competent provider, but only the smallest fraction of HCWs can meet that standard, and the rest have no particular interest in acknowledging this. It is too hard to expect each HCW (or any of the rest of us) to inform potential patients that others are more skillful. It is hard enough for any of us even to know the limits of our competency.

That HIV-positive HCWs would be hesitant to reveal this information should not be surprising. It is clear that once infection with HIV is announced, patients will flee. (Is this flight caused by informed choice or irrational fear?) As Gostin has pointed out, because patients will desert an HIV-positive HCW, revealing this information to patients is tantamount to accepting the (illegal) discrimination that occurs as a result.[26]

Some final implications of the notion that patients should have the ultimate power to determine what is informed consent are troubling. Consider the HIV-positive HCW (say, a psychiatrist) who presents *no* threat of infecting patients through medical care. What if a patient nevertheless demands to know the provider's HIV status as a condition of care. Must the HCW disclose it even though once that knowledge becomes public, most patients will choose to go elsewhere? If the patient is the only one who determines the conditions of informed consent, then the answer must be yes. The experts might reply that such disclosure provides no useful information for the patient and, as a response to irrational fear, need not be offered. Yet patients might respond that as their "comfort" with the provider is a most important part of the healing process, this information is essential for making them comfortable.

Bergalis, for her part, also feared the consequences of making her infection known publicly and initially sought to conceal this information from others. Indeed, Bergalis did not disclose the fact that she had AIDS to a dentist who treated her.[27] When asked why she did not tell the dentist, Bergalis replied,

> Well, I had read about other families that were burned out of their homes and, and I was just extremely scared and I didn't know how the neighbors were going to react or how the dental office was going to react, if they would kick me out or . . . if somebody was going to scream. . . . I didn't know what kind of reaction I was going to have.[28]

It is perhaps easy to sympathize with the demands of the Bergalis family and other patients for testing, restrictions, and disclosure. But it is also worth considering these issues from the eyes of an infected provider. Health care workers are humans, too, and they—at least the infected ones—also have personal reasons to oppose the policies that the Bergalises sought. In the words of one anonymous family practitioner,

> My patients like me, love me, depend on me. But if they find out I have HIV, why should they be crusaders? They won't. . . . If there was the slightest possibility I could give it to them it would be their right to know I'm HIV-positive. But there is no conceivable way. So it is absolutely not their business. . . .
>
> I know much more today about what it means to be a good doctor. God, do I know now what it's like to have a doctor listen to you. When you are frightened, helpless, and in need of guidance, it's a marvelous feeling to have someone work with you to make you better. Let me tell you, it's a miracle to find someone to help you.[29]

There are no simple answers to the questions of what HCWs must tell their patients. We should be uneasy with the idea that experts are the only ones who should decide what information HCWs must disclose. But we should also be troubled by the notion that HCWs must reveal whatever patients demand.

DIFFICULT ISSUES

Whether or not there should be mandatory testing, practice restrictions, and patient notification were individually difficult questions. They were not, however, entirely separate ones, and the relationship among them made developing policy even more troublesome. Patient notification was only justified, it was argued, if the risks were substantial. Yet if the risks were substantial, it is hard to see how notifying patients alone would be enough; substantial risks call for practice restrictions.[30] And if risks were large enough to require practice restrictions, then why just have voluntary testing? If the risks of infection were trivial, then notification, restrictions, and testing were all unwarranted; if the risks were grave, then all three policies were needed.

These issues would be difficult to resolve even in an environment of mutual respect. Unfortunately, it is always tempting to believe that your preferences are the "correct" ones and that those who disagree with you are ignorant, foolish, or evil. So it was here. Patients, at least as exemplified by the Bergalises, were at times inclined to view medical professionals not as unbiased authorities but as a special interest group determined to protect its position. Accordingly, those who opposed the patients' recommendations must do so only because they wanted to protect their own privacy, privileges, and pocketbooks. Meanwhile, many experts seemed to see patients as making absurd demands about matters of which they knew little and understood less.

The Bergalis family was radical not by seeking extreme changes in policy but in its vision of what was possible in America. This vision put the ordinary individual first. The patient, not the medical establishment, should be supreme in deciding what risks are acceptable in the medical setting and what kind of information the patient should receive. Moreover, the citizen, not the public health officials, should be sovereign in determining what health policy should be. Most strikingly, the Bergalis family believed that a single individual—Kimberly—could inspire these changes in medical care and public policy.

Thoughtful experts were sympathetic with the idea that the patient, not the medical provider, should be the one who ultimately makes decisions about what kind of care is appropriate and in what circumstances this care should be delivered. Yet there was also deep concern about creating a medical system in which patient fears could prevail, especially if this meant that others—in this case, the HIV-positive HCW—would needlessly suffer even more than they already did, without clear benefit to public health. Experts thus had their own radical view: public health policies should be based on evidence, not fear. They wanted patients who were not quite sovereign.

The policy questions all involved complex ethical and practical considerations, but they consequently also involved one strictly empirical one: the risk of HIV infection in the medical workplace. The higher these risks, the greater the merits of testing, restricting, and notifying; the lower the risks, the less the merits. Patients and experts might well disagree about how much risk was too much, of course, but without data concerning the size of the risk these disagreements would remain purely conjectural.

RISKS OF INFECTION

The CDC was thus vitally interested in estimating the probability that a patient would contract HIV from an HCW while receiving medical care. There were two main ways it could do this. The first used the actual number of persons infected and the actual number of HCWs (or infected HCWs or infected dentists, for example). The CDC did not see this method as very useful, as Acer has accounted for all the known patient infections. Excluding Acer, the apparent probability that a patient would contract HIV while receiving medical care seemed to be zero.

A second method of estimating the risk of infection, and the one the CDC used, was to identify the steps necessary for an infection to occur and then to calculate the risk based on the probability of each step happening.

For a patient to be accidentally infected with HIV by an HCW in the medical setting, four things had to happen: (1) the HCW had to be infected; (2) the HCW had to suffer an injury severe enough to expose blood; (3) the blood had to come into contact with the patient's blood; and (4) the virus actually had to spread to the patient. The likelihood that any patient would be infected during any procedure depended on the chance that all four things happened. Furthermore, if one knew how many HCWs were infected, how often they cut themselves and exposed these cuts to their patients' blood, and how often infections occurred as a result, one could estimate the total number of patients around the country that were likely to be infected by their HCWs. The main problem was that, at the time it was reconsidering the HIV guidelines, the CDC did not know *any* of these numbers or probabilities. The CDC did not know how many HCWs were infected, how often HCWs injured themselves while providing patient care, how frequently these injuries came into contact with patients' blood, or how common infection was if contact occurred.

As a result, the CDC had to estimate—that is, guess—each of the individual probabilities. Because the overall risk of infection depends on the individual probabilities, the uncertainties at each step become magnified, leading to great uncertainty about the overall risk. The CDC nonetheless attempted in January 1991 to estimate the risk of HIV transmission in the health care setting and the number of patients likely to be infected.[31] Here is a brief summary of its analysis.

Little data existed on HCW injury rates; the CDC was able to cite just six fairly small studies that examined surgical or obstetrical injury rates.[32] These studies showed that injury rates varied by specialty, procedure, location, and especially by individual. The CDC itself had conducted one study in four hospitals where 1,382 surgical procedures were watched; injuries were reported in 88 (2.5 percent) of the procedures.[33] No such studies had been published concerning injury rates by dentists; the CDC thus *assumed* that dentists cut themselves less frequently, assigning them a 0.4 percent chance of self-injury during a procedure. In the hospital study, 28 of the injuries resulted in recontact with the patient; recontact was thus observed in 32 percent (28 of 88) of the injuries. Most (75 percent) of these 28 recontacts involved suture needles. The CDC then *assumed* that the dentists who injured themselves had the same recontact rates as those in surgery, 32 percent.

Even less was known about the frequency with which HCWs transmitted HIV to their patients. Three "look-back" (retrospective) studies had not found any patients infected by three HIV-positive surgeons.[34] Several other studies had documented that HCWs had themselves been infected through occupational exposure; these studies suggested that 0.3 percent of HCWs exposed to a single needlestick from an HIV-infected needle contracted the virus.[35] A much larger number of studies had implicated certain invasive surgical and dental procedures in transmitting hepatitis to patients.[36] These studies suggested that 30 percent of those similarly exposed to the hepatitis B virus became infected. Yet the relevance of these studies was open to question, given the small number of hepatitis outbreaks that occurred when universal precautions were followed and the estimate that the risk of transmitting HIV may be one hundred times less than that of transmitting hepatitis. The CDC nonetheless guessed that between 0.3 and 0.003 percent of patients exposed to HIV by HCWs with minor injuries would become infected.

Using these slender data and best guesses, the CDC thus estimated that the risk of contracting HIV from an infected dentist was between 1 in 263,000 (0.0000038) and 1 in 2,630,000 (0.00000038). (This risk is calculated from injury rate times recontact rate times infection rate:

$$0.004 \times 0.32 \times 0.003 = .0000038$$

The estimated probability that a patient of an HIV-infected surgeon would be infected during surgery was between 1 in 42,000 (0.0024) and 1 in 417,000 (0.00024). These calculations suggested to the CDC that HIV-positive HCWs had already infected between ten and one hundred other patients.[37] The basis for the estimates regarding HIV transmission was shaky, to say the least. Still, this was the best that could be done at the time, given the paucity of data. (Since then, about twenty thousand patients of HIV-positive physicians have been studied; it appears that none of these patients were infected by their medical provider.)

It is quite difficult to put these risks into context.[38] One possible way is to compare the probability of HIV infection in the health care setting with other risks that patients face. It has been estimated that five out of every one hundred thousand patients die from other infections contracted while they are in a hospital, for example, while ten die from complications associated with anesthesia, seventeen die from complications during or after vaginal deliveries, fifty die from complications during or after an unnecessary operation, and one hundred die from complications during or after a hysterectomy.[39] Because all these medical treatments create much higher rates than those posed by HIV-positive HCWs, most experts have concluded that patients were overreacting to the threat of AIDS and that the risks were not high enough to merit strong action.

But evaluating risks is not merely a matter of toting up objective probabilities. It is clear that for most people, subjective concerns are also critically important. Individuals are more concerned about risks that are involuntary (such as unknowingly being treated by an HIV-positive HCW) rather than voluntary (such as agreeing to undergo anesthesia). Individuals worry about risks that can cause particularly odious consequences; death from anesthesia might be seen as far preferable to death from AIDS. Thus, it is perfectly rational for individuals to place greater emphasis on controlling certain rare risks than on controlling other more common ones.

These were extraordinarily difficult problems, and no group had a monopoly on satisfactory answers. The guidelines of the American Medical Association (AMA) came the closest to those advocated by patients regarding HIV and HCWs—and the AMA came under withering criticism from other experts as a result. Even before Bergalis, the AMA guidelines in 1988 read that "patients are entitled to expect that their physician will not increase their exposure to the risk of contracting an infectious disease, even *minimally*. . . . If a risk does exist, the physician should not engage in the activity."[40] The AMA reiterated this policy in 1991 when it proclaimed that HIV-infected physicians "have an ethical obligation not to engage in any professional practice which has an *identifiable* risk of transmission to patients." [41]

These statements have been ridiculed by other experts. In a typical example, Mark Barnes, at that time the policy director of the New York

State AIDS Institute, pointed out that such a "no identifiable risk" standard would be impossible for any HCW to attain, as every HCW creates some risk of infecting patients (through, if nothing else, the "indigenous microflora" we all carry) or otherwise damaging them through conditions (such as aging, stress, fatigue, marital problems, psychiatric treatment, medication side effects, drug or alcohol use) that create even more readily identifiable risks than HIV infection.[42]

TWO STRATEGIES

The conflict between patients and experts left the CDC in a difficult position. In their heads, CDC officials *were* the experts, and this perspective was their own. In their hearts, the CDC officials recognized the merit of the public's opinion and gave voice to it during their policy deliberations. They also knew that if they ignored the public they might well place their organization in jeopardy, yet if they appeared to pander to mass sentiment, their medical credentials would be tarnished. Although not directly controlled by the public, the CDC was supervised by Congress (through its appropriations and oversight functions). If the CDC did not take the steps necessary to calm public fear, Congress might force it to do so. And while not directly dependent on the medical community for support, the CDC could not operate effectively unless HCWs believed in its efforts.

The CDC officials might also be forgiven if they saw no obvious way to satisfy patient and expert concerns. The policy goals of these groups seemed to be largely incompatible: HCWs are either required to be tested or they are not; HIV-positive HCWs either must notify their patients or they need not. If the CDC adopted the public's preferences, it would reject those of the experts, and vice versa.

The CDC could attempt to resolve these conflicts through either "substantive" or "procedural" moves. In the first instance, the CDC could attempt to develop public health recommendations that resolved the apparent contradictions and met the policy concerns of both the public and the professionals. In the second, the CDC could adopt some set of methods that would allow it to make policy decisions that might settle the disagreements.

Procedural methods to resolve conflict indeed are at the heart of our nation's political and legal systems. The genius of democracy and the wisdom of the law are that they establish methods—such as campaigns and elections, or jury trials—that allow the various interests to make their claims and then allow decisions to be based on these claims. Elections and trials do not, of course, guarantee that all sides will be satisfied with the results; the goal is simply that the participants will view the results as legitimate because the process used to arrive at them was fair. Unfortunately, the more passionately the participants hold a belief, the less likely it is that they will accept as fair a decision that rejects their position. While the CDC could use procedural methods to help resolve the conflict between the professionals and the public, it could by no means ensure that these methods would secure consensus.

Moreover, the situation the CDC faced was not entirely analogous to those existing during elections and trials. Elections, after all, are ultimately about popularity in the choice among competing persons or proposals; whoever gets the most votes is, by democratic definition, the best candidate. (It does not make sense, however, to think of any candidate as the "correct" one.) Trials, in contrast, are finally about truth: a person is either innocent or guilty of breaking the law, and it is the task of the judge and jury to discover this truth. Courts, in theory, can actually identify correct answers.

The CDC, in developing its public health recommendations, was neither conducting an electoral popularity contest nor a legal discovery of the truth. The CDC could not justify its decisions on the grounds that they were either correct or popular. Elections and trials are not easy, but the CDC faced an even tougher task. To maintain its legitimacy with the citizenry, the CDC had to devise health guidelines that at least were not widely protested or, better yet, were broadly supported as truly protecting public health. To maintain its credibility with the medical community, the CDC needed to choose policies that met scientific standards of efficacy. Ideally, these policies would have public health benefits known to be larger than their side effects. The substantive strategy would be for the CDC to devise recommendations with content acceptable to both the public and the professionals. While the policy preferences of these groups were apparently contradictory, there was still the slim possibility that the CDC could define a position acceptable to popular opinion and scientific evidence. In the year after the Bergalis case was made public, the CDC pursued both procedural and substantive angles. Neither proved easy, as we shall see in the next chapter.

CHAPTER SIX

Politics

The CDC's Guidelines

I

n one sense, Bergalis's claim that the government had "stood by not doing a damn thing" about the risk of AIDS transmission was correct. There were no laws specifically protecting patients from health care workers who had AIDS. On the other hand, the CDC had not exactly just been standing by. CDC officials had long been aware that HIV could be spread among patients and their health care providers and had taken steps to prevent this from happening. Indeed, before Bergalis was diagnosed with AIDS, the CDC had already issued seven sets of guidelines concerning HIV in the health care setting.[1]

BEFORE THE ACER CASE

Initially, however, these guidelines were mainly concerned with protecting health care workers (HCWs) from their patients. This did not mean that the CDC was more concerned with protecting the lives of doctors than those of the sick; it merely recognized that HCWs were more likely to be infected by patients than vice versa. By the time the Bergalis case was announced, the CDC had reported that perhaps forty HCWs had been infected with HIV through accidental contact with patients' blood.[2]

Still, the evolution of the CDC's guidelines on this reveal the CDC's uncertainty about what measures would best protect the public health.[3] The 1985 recommendations indicated that

> a risk of transmission of [HIV] infection from HCWs to patients would exist in situations where there is both (1) a high degree of trauma to the patient that would provide a portal of entry for the virus (e.g., during invasive procedures) and (2) access of blood or serous fluid from the infected HCW to the open tissue of the patient, as would occur if the HCW sustained a needlestick or scalpel injury during an invasive procedure.[4]

The recommendations went further to suggest that HIV-infected HCWs who performed no invasive procedures need not be restricted further; however, the CDC noted that it was considering "whether additional restrictions are indicated for HCWs who perform invasive procedures." In either case, HCWs known to be infected were advised to consult with their personal physicians and employers to determine work assignments that would best protect the HCW's health. The CDC also stated that there was no basis for routinely conducting HIV tests for those HCWs who performed only noninvasive procedures but noted that it was considering "whether the indications exist for [HIV] testing of HCWs who perform invasive procedures."[5] Finally, the CDC emphasized that all HCWs should use universal precautions whenever dealing with blood or other potentially infectious bodily fluids. "Universal precautions" are those actions, such as washing hands, wearing gloves and masks, using and disposing needles and other sharp instruments properly, and disinfecting and sterilizing instruments, that are designed to prevent the spread of infectious diseases.[6]

In the 1986 guidelines the CDC reiterated how important universal precautions were for preventing the spread of all infectious diseases, and it provided much more specific advice on how to follow these precautions. The CDC then went further than it had in 1985 in rejecting the concept of mandatory testing or practice restrictions. The CDC argued—in contrast to its ambivalence the previous year—that testing HCWs who performed invasive procedures was "not necessary . . . since the risk of transmission [of HIV] in this setting is so low"; mandatory screening "would not practically supplement" universal precautions in "further reducing the negligible risk of transmission" from HIV-infected HCWs to patients. Infected HCWs could thus continue providing all types of treatment so long as they properly used universal precautions.[7]

By 1987 the CDC again was less than certain about some of these conclusions. The guidelines issued in that year gave the fateful message that "although transmission of HIV from infected health care workers to patients has not been reported, transmission during invasive procedures remains a possibility."[8] The CDC reminded its readers, however, that the transmission of HIV from HCW to patient would "occur only very rarely, if at all." The CDC still maintained that HCWs who follow universal precautions "will minimize" the risk of transmission.[9]

Yet given that a theoretical possibility of transmission existed, the CDC no longer rejected mandatory HIV testing out-of-hand. Instead, the CDC now suggested that "the utility of routine testing of . . . HCWs to prevent transmission of HIV cannot be assessed." Before it could be assessed "the frequency of testing, as well as the issues of consent, confidentiality, and consequences of test results . . . must be addressed."[10] The CDC continued to reject explicitly the general rule that HIV-positive HCWs should be prohibited from providing medical care:

> The question of whether workers infected with HIV—especially those who perform invasive procedures—can adequately and safely be allowed to perform patient-care duties or whether their work assignments should be changed *must* be determined on an individual basis [emphasis added]. These decisions should be made by the HCW's personal physician(s) in conjunction with the medical directors and personnel health service staff of the employing institution or hospital.[11]

Note that two subtle changes had crept in from the previous year's recommendations. Now the CDC implied that all HCWs infected with HIV—not just those performing invasive procedures—should be assessed to determine whether they could safely provide care. Moreover, by indicating that some HCWs might not be able to provide patient care safely, the CDC is tacitly admitting that universal precautions might not be enough to prevent transmission.

Still, what remained unstated became most heatedly debated. None of the 1985, 1986, and 1987 recommendations mentioned "patient notification." The idea that HIV-positive HCWs should disclose their diagnosis to their patients before treating them is simply not discussed.

The CDC had developed these guidelines as a routine part of its mission to protect the public health. In quieter times, the CDC wrote its public health recommendations by assembling the relevant experts (doctors, epidemiologists, and other infection control specialists), who would, out of the glare of the public spotlight, draw up the recommendations based on their best understanding of medical prevention. Producing recommendations, therefore, was mainly a process of developing a consensus among experts. The CDC did not produce its recommendations on any fixed schedule, but instead wrote and revised them as deemed necessary by the experts based on such factors as changes in knowledge about health risks or infection control. When the working group of experts had finished, the recommendations were published in the *MMWR* without the imprimatur of the CDC as a whole.

The CDC's recommendations, while influential within the medical community, were not official policy of the Department of Health and Human Services (HHS), nor were they legally binding. (The CDC can recommend that its guidelines become a "standard of care," however, and courts have often given these standards great weight in medical malpractice suits.) In bureaucratic terms, this means that the CDC did not have to follow the Administrative Procedures Act (APA) in writing them.[12] The APA requires federal agencies, when they are writing new regulations, to follow certain methods. The key provisions (found in APA section 533) dictate that before federal agencies issue regulations, they must publish the proposed rule in the *Federal Register* (including "a statement of the time, place, and nature of the public rule making proceedings"), must provide for a public comment period of at least thirty days on the proposed rule, and must provide any interested person the right to petition "for the issuance, amendment, or repeal of the rule."[13] Because the CDC did not have to follow these procedures when it wrote its recommendations, the public was effectively cut out of the process by which the early versions of the HIV recommendations were developed.

The fact that the CDC was not obliged to consider public comments in issuing its recommendations had certain obvious advantages, at least from the perspective of the agency. Freedom from the APA meant that the CDC's public health experts could develop guidelines without having to pay direct attention to the concerns of interest groups or popular opinion. Without public interference, these experts could write recommendations more quickly and based more heavily on medical evidence than on partisan pressure, interest group lobbying, or public sentiments.

Yet these professional advantages were also political handicaps. Without public involvement, the CDC's recommendations could hardly presume to be responsive to public concerns. Without popular review of and comment on proposed recommendations, the nation's citizens might understandably be skeptical of claims that the CDC worked in their interest. These handicaps would be minor if the experts always did what the public wanted and if the public always wanted what the experts did. Such fortunate circumstances were usually the rule before the onset of AIDS: the public wanted infections to be controlled, and public health officials gave them infection control. But AIDS changed the rules. On this issue, as on many others involving this disease, the opinions of patients and experts were often quite different.

STRUGGLING TO RESOLVE THE CONFLICTS

At the moment that Curran, Jaffe, Ciesielski, and other CDC officials concluded that Acer had infected Bergalis, they knew that the CDC would face pressure to rewrite its recommendations regarding HIV and HCWs. It would simply be unacceptable—medically and politically—for the CDC to have told the public, "Fear not. You are already safe." As Jaffe noted, "we could not just [truthfully] say 'Well, this is a one-in-a-million happening, so let's not worry.'"[14]

On August 13 and 14, 1990, slightly more than two weeks after the *MMWR* announced the case and two weeks before Acer released his letter to the public, the CDC held a first "consultants" meeting to discuss revising its HIV recommendations.[15] The purpose of this meeting was not to rewrite the recommendations—or even to develop a consensus regarding them—but to raise the main questions, to develop a common understanding of the issues, and to identify areas of conflict.

Almost sixty organizations from outside the federal government, plus representatives from at least eighteen universities and seven state health departments, as well as ten federal agencies and some twenty CDC officials attended this by-invitation meeting. (A list of the attending organizations appears in Appendix Three.) The experts were heavily represented. Health care organizations from the American Academy of Family Physicians to the United States Conference of Local Health Officers attended, as did the largest and most prominent ones, the American Medical Association and the American Dental Association. The participants were also highly professional in their credentials: the room was filled with forty-eight doctors, sixteen professors, seven dentists, seven nurses, and at least six persons with other graduate degrees; many participants also listed other degrees. Still, at least ten organizations present were not composed of health care professionals, and one group (the National Society for Patient Representation and Consumer Affairs) was, at least by its title, specifically dedicated to assisting patients. This was not a meeting of ordinary patients, however; only seven participants did not list an advanced degree.

This meeting was thus dominated by highly educated professionals primarily serving as delegates of medical interest groups. That the participants looked nothing like the public as a whole will not surprise students of American politics. In the United States, even more than in other countries, citizens with higher socioeconomic status are likelier to engage in all forms of political participation than those with less education, wealth, and prestige.[16] Organized interest groups often dominate agency hearings, at least numerically, while participation by the public is typically smaller and more sporadic. Still, groups representing the public can and do influence bureaucratic decision making, especially when public officials are already sympathetic to the public interest.[17]

By all accounts, the CDC did not come to this meeting with firm ideas about either the problems or the solutions. Indeed, when questioned as to whether the CDC planned to impose restrictions on HIV-positive HCWs, Curran answered, "That's the purpose of the whole meeting: we don't have a fixed CDC view, yet."[18] The CDC officials did come, however, with the belief that the views of both experts and patients were important. In defense of the expert view, Curran argued that "we aren't going to make recommendations for public relations purposes, but only if there is scientific justification. If there's no evidence of risk, we shouldn't be making recommendations in this area. Our credibility doesn't depend just on the public, but also our colleagues."[19]

Curran did recognize the importance of public opinion, however. For example, the CDC's existing recommendations called for HCWs infected with the hepatitis B virus (a sometimes fatal disease) to have their practices restricted only *after* they had infected a patient. In considering whether the CDC should have similar policies for HCW with HIV, Curran stated, "That would not be acceptable to people."[20] Similarly, Jaffe argued on behalf of patients by asserting, "If we created a straw consumer who was listening to this [discussion], he would say that if there was an infected person who might expose me to infection, he should not work on me. If we pointed out that this would lead to testing, he might say, 'That's OK with me.'"[21]

This meeting was not designed to produce a consensus, and, in this, it succeeded. During the next four months, then, the CDC continued its internal deliberations. Nothing about them was easy. The issues were difficult enough, but the political environment added another layer of complexity. Some medical organizations were wary of the project because they remained skeptical that Bergalis had even been infected by her dentist. As Jaffe put it,

> The dental and medical professions were very ambivalent about the Acer case. At the beginning, they wanted to pretend it hadn't happened. The ADA [American Dental Association] and AMA [American Medical Association] had to be dragged very reluctantly into the process of designing some kind of guidelines to make sure that this didn't happen again.[22]

But if the ADA and AMA were reluctant to work with the CDC, other organizations were unwilling to be left out of the process. Shortly after the consultants meeting, the American Civil Liberties Union (concerned that the CDC was moving toward a policy of testing and restrictions) sent a letter to the general counsel of the Department of Health and Human Services, claiming that the CDC was violating the law by rushing to develop public policy in private. (Despite the large number of organizations present at the consultants meeting, it was not advertised as open to the public.) David Rogers, the cochair of the National AIDS Commission, concurred that the CDC was moving too quickly and urged CDC director William Roper, HHS assistant secretary James Mason (Roper's boss and Rogers's good friend), and HHS secretary Louis Sullivan to move forward more judiciously.[23]

Roper, an experienced political adviser and bureaucrat, was persuaded. Although he was fairly new to the CDC, he had served previously as the director of the Health Care Financing Administration

(HCFA, which is responsible for administering the Medicare and Medicaid programs) and on the Domestic Policy Council within the Reagan and Bush White Houses. Whether he was influenced by his experience with the HCFA (which is bound by the rules of the Administrative Procedures Act) or by the letter from the ACLU, Roper decided that his next step would be to hold a formal public meeting "to assess the risk of HIV and hepatitis infection during invasive [medical] procedures and to determine the appropriate response."[24] The time (February 21 and 22, 1991), place (the Hyatt Regency Hotel in Atlanta), and conditions (seating limited to one thousand) were duly advertised in the *Federal Register*.[25]

This meeting was even larger than the first, with approximately one hundred groups, together with other individuals, participating. Echoing the August gathering, Roper pledged that "we are here to listen," that "we don't have a fixed, made-up mind on what to do from here on this subject," and that "we'll not expect to reach a consensus within . . . this meeting."[26] Again, Roper's expectations were almost completely met.

While the two-day meeting produced some agreements—for example, virtually all participants except Kuvin, the medical adviser to the Bergalis family, opposed mandatory testing—it also generated a wide variety of perspectives (and a transcript of almost five hundred pages) regarding risks and recommendations. It also raised a couple of extremely knotty problems for the CDC regarding the relevant facts and their interpretation. All the major issues—what were the risks, should HIV-positive HCWs be restricted, should they notify their patients—were aired but left unresolved.

The participants agreed that public health guidelines needed to be based on data concerning the risks of HIV transmission. HCWs who did not pose any real risks of transmitting HIV to their patients should not be restricted from providing care; those who did pose real risks should be restricted. The participants did not agree, however, about who posed risks, how large these risks were, and what the restrictions should be.

There were almost no data to help. By the time of the meeting, the CDC had determined that at least four of Acer's patients had been infected while receiving medical care. No other cases of HCWs transmitting HIV to patients had been documented, and four additional investigations of HIV-positive HCWs (involving three surgeons and one dentist) found no other instances of transmission from HCW to patient. In reviewing this evidence, the CDC's David Bell, chief of AIDS activity in the Hospital Infections Program, forthrightly acknowledged that the existing studies were quite limited and that "it seems unlikely that more precise estimates of patient risk will be available . . . in the near future."[27]

Using the scanty data, Bell nonetheless presented the CDC's imprecise estimates. According to its best guesses, the probability that a patient of an HIV-infected surgeon would be infected during surgery was between 1 in 42,000 and 1 in 417,000; the risk of being infected by an HIV-positive dentist was much lower, between 1 in 263,000 and 1 in 2,630,000.[28]

These estimates were alternately attacked and belittled. Even with these minute risks, the ADA argued that the CDC had greatly overestimated the probability of infection; the ADA's estimates were only half as high as the CDC's.[29] Other participants pointed out that these models could not begin to explain the Acer practice, where four (and ultimately six) one-in-a-million events apparently occurred. One speaker, noting that in fact no surgeons had been implicated in infecting patients, wondered sarcastically when the CDC was going to develop a statistical evaluation of the risk of HIV infection from "mosquitoes, toilet seats, or waiters."[30]

The CDC, for its part, recognized all these criticisms. No, Bell acknowledged, the CDC did not know whether these probabilities were accurate. Time and again, Bell responded to questions by agreeing, "We don't know what the risk is," and to criticisms by conceding, "These are the data we have."[31] Even the mosquito remark was dignified by what must have been an aggravated Curran:

I think that is a very important comment. A risk assessment model is inherently risky . . . [but it] is an attempt also to try to put this in some perspective; in a situation when we know the risk is not zero, to say to the public this risk we think falls within these kind of logical bounds, and we want to change these bounds with any data we can get or any theory we can get.[32]

Unfortunately, obtaining the data necessary to make precise estimates would be expensive, time consuming, and controversial. Researchers would need to identify many HIV-infected HCWs, contact their patients, test them for HIV, and investigate their behavioral risk. Since the risk of transmission was known to be fairly low, estimating the risk with any precision would mean that many thousands of patients would need to be investigated. As Bell noted, "even if all patients in a large study are [HIV] negative, we cannot statistically exclude the possibility that transmission could occur at a low rate."[33] If the risk of infection were truly one in a million, the implication is that a million patients would have to be investigated to find just one who was infected. Yet without clear knowledge about the magnitude of the risk, it seemed impossible to know if it was large enough to justify restricting infected practitioners or requiring them to reveal their infection to their patients. The ACLU—this time, inside the room—also reminded the audience, "Any guidelines [the CDC] promulgates in this area must be consistent with applicable legal principles"—that is, with the Americans with Disabilities Act.[34]

The shortage of data concerning HIV transmission by HCWs created a central dilemma for the CDC. Without data, the CDC had no "scientific" basis for changing its policies. But the public was hardly of the opinion that more data should be collected—if data meant "more infections." The experts wanted data before action, while patients wanted action before data.

Roper closed the meeting by reminding the participants that this had only been "one step in a careful and deliberative process" of developing guidelines. He outlined the next steps (which bore a striking resemblance to formal regulatory proceedings):

> Following this two-day meeting, written comments may be submitted to CDC within thirty days. Then we will develop draft recommendations, taking into consideration the comments and information available at that time. The draft recommendations will be released for a further sixty-day period before final recommendations are issued.[35]

The "then" took a long time. Throughout the spring of 1991, the CDC, in consultation with other public health officials within HHS and experts outside the department, did develop numerous drafts of the proposed recommendations. (Jaffe once claimed that the number of drafts had moved into triple digits.[36]) But the sharp divisions within the agency regarding the content of—or even the need for—revised recommendations stalled the CDC. The difficult questions raised at the open meeting were not easy for the agency to answer.

One can sense the scrutiny received by each phrase and every word. A draft dated March 25 lists several "exposure-prone invasive procedures"—those presumably that created some risk of transmitting HIV.[37] By April 5 the wording had been changed to "*potentially* exposure-prone invasive procedures" (emphasis added).[38] Apparently, someone had argued convincingly that it had not been demonstrated that any procedures were *conclusively* prone to exposure.

Broader disagreements were also manifest. In the March 25 draft, the CDC suggested that "HCWs who are infected with HIV or HBV and who perform invasive procedures not identified as exposure-prone should consult with their personal physician(s) regarding whether they can safely perform patient care duties or whether their work assignments should be changed."[39] Less than two weeks later, the CDC had changed its mind and now found that "currently available data provide no basis for recommendations for restricting the practice of HCWs infected with HIV or HBV who perform invasive procedures not identified as exposure-prone."[40]

CDC officials remained stuck, wanting to make new recommendations but lacking new data on which to build them.

The April 5, 1991, memo from Roper to Mason presenting and discussing possible recommendations is instructive. This memo presented four options, with pros and cons listed for each. The first, to maintain the status quo, was presented with little discussion. Option 2 recommended against restricting HIV-positive HCWs and proposed vigorous adherence to universal precautions, as well as close monitoring of the situation for additional developments. The major pluses given for this option were that it was the least intrusive and easiest to implement. A long list of cons followed. It was noted that additional HIV infections may occur even if universal precautions are used, that better data about risks would not be available for a long time, and that the CDC would need, as it put it, "rapidly to reevaluate" the recommendation when additional cases of infection were documented.

Option 3 called for mandatory testing of HCWs who performed certain procedures and restricting those HCWs who tested positive for HIV or HBV. The benefits of this recommendation were seen mainly in administrative terms: it could be implemented uniformly, and it eased the burden of decision making by creating a hard-and-fast rule. (It is revealing that "reducing infection" is *not* listed as a plus.) The negatives, again, loomed larger. Testing and restricting would be expensive, difficult to administer, intrusive, and not entirely effective.

The fourth option was the one the agency favored. It emphasized "professional responsibility" in recommending that HCWs who performed certain procedures should learn their HIV status and, if they were infected, refrain from performing these procedures. This narrow and limited recommendation was preferred because it was judged to take actions that were commensurate with the risks. Still, the CDC recognized that this option could lead to inadequate and inconsistent compliance and that "public perception of risk reduction will not be as high as in Option 3."[41]

While the CDC was struggling to develop new guidelines, the issue of what to do about HCWs with AIDS again became highly visible to the public. On June 14, 1991, the CDC released yet another update on the Bergalis case, indicating now that at least five patients had contracted HIV from Acer while receiving dental treatment from him.[42] On that same day, Philip Benson, an obstetrician-gynecologist in Minneapolis, notified 328 of his patients that he had AIDS and recommended that they receive HIV tests. After this case became widely publicized, one of Benson's colleagues publicly announced that he also had AIDS.[43] On June 24, during a press conference at the American Medical Association's annual meeting, Vice President Quayle stated that HCWs should be required to take HIV tests and disclose the results to their patients.[44] On June 28, 1991, the day before he died, a dentist in North Carolina notified his patients that he had AIDS.[45] On the first of July, *Newsweek*'s cover story was entitled "Doctors with AIDS."[46] Inside, a two-page photo showed the dying Bergalis, and the article included a reprint of her open, angry letter to Economou.[47] (As Bergalis mailed this letter to the press rather than to Economou and other health officials, they first read about it in the media, just as Kimberly had first heard her case announced on national television. In response to Bergalis's letter, Florida's public health offices were swamped with angry phone calls and letters.) *Newsweek* also reported the results of a poll showing that 90 percent of the respondents agreed that all HCWs with the AIDS virus should be required to tell their patients.[48]

CONGRESS FORCES THE ISSUE

Motivated by these stories, Congress—or at least a couple of prominent conservative members of Congress—prepared to take action.[49] Representative Robert Dannemeyer from California, ranking Republican on the House Energy and Commerce Committee, a well-known homophobe and a "persistent critic of the CDC and the entire public health establishment," acted first by introducing the "Kimberly Bergalis Patient and Health Providers' Protection Act of 1991" on June 26.[50] This legislation required that all health care workers who performed invasive procedures be tested for HIV and hepatitis, and it prohibited infected HCWs from performing any invasive procedures unless the patient expressly approved it.[51] Senator Dole, the leader of the Republican Party in the Senate, also believed that a decisive response was needed to calm the public and planned to submit a measure requiring patient notification. HHS secretary Sullivan personally called the senator to persuade him to wait until the CDC guidelines were released before acting.[52]

Shortly after introducing his bill, Dannemeyer personally invited Kimberly to testify on the Bergalis Act before the Health and Environment Subcommittee on September 10. A formal invitation was slow in arriving, however, and the Bergalis family began to suspect that her appearance was being delayed by opponents of the bill in the hope that she would be too ill to testify. Tim Westmoreland, a staffer for Henry A. Waxman (D–California and chair of the committee), finally called the Bergalis family to tell them that the hearing had been postponed; he encouraged Bergalis to submit her comments in writing. Mr. Bergalis, who by now had numerous contacts in the media, spread the word that Waxman was trying to prevent Kimberly from appearing before Congress. Westmoreland again called the Bergalis family, assuring them that the committee wanted Kimberly to appear. He invited her to testify on September 19, but Mr. Bergalis insisted that that was too soon (given Kimberly's failing health). "Look," he said. "My daughter is dying. In fact, we think the only reason she's still alive is to make sure she gets her say before your bureaucrats. She deserves that before she dies. We need time to make sure she is ready for the trip."[53] The hearing was rescheduled for September 26, 1991.

On Thursday, July 11, Senator Jesse Helms (R–North Carolina), the self-proclaimed "most radical person" regarding AIDS, raised the stakes by submitting Amendment 734 to the bill appropriating funds for the Treasury and other agencies, declaring that HIV-positive health care workers who did not reveal their diagnosis to patients before treating them were subject to $10,000 fines or ten years in prison.[54] Helms rejected criticisms that this amendment was too punitive. Health care workers with AIDS who continue to practice "should be treated no better than the criminal who guns down a helpless victim on the street."[55] Quoting Bergalis's open letter that called such health care providers bastards, Helms added, "That is exactly what they are. No, that is a reflection on bastards, to call them bastards. They are worse than that."[56]

Not eager to abdicate its responsibility for public health to elected politicians (or to send doctors to jail), the CDC rushed to release its own HIV guidelines. In contrast to the legislation pending in Congress, which sought universal and mandatory HIV testing for HCWs, mandatory patient notification, and criminal sanctions to bolster these mandates, the CDC's latest proposal endorsed limited and voluntary action by HCWs. According to this CDC draft, HCWs who performed certain procedures (not limited to invasive ones but still only those that were "exposure-prone") "should know" their HIV status and should seek counsel from expert review panels regarding their fitness to provide medical treatment. On Friday, July 12, the CDC sent its recommendations to the printer.

At the last minute, when the proof version of the CDC's guidelines was ready for printing, Senator Orrin Hatch (R–Utah) asked to be briefed on the recommendations by HHS secretary Louis Sullivan.[57] At this meeting Hatch asked Sullivan to add a provision to the guidelines stating that HIV-positive HCWs *would* notify patients of this before providing them care. The secretary agreed to make the change. The proofs were pulled from the printer, an eighteen-word sentence involving patient notification was inserted, and the recommendations were published (see Appendix Four). As Hatch justified the change:

> The American people support health care professionals disclosing this information to their patients. Over 90 percent of our citizens support mandatory disclosure by nurses, physicians, and dentists who are infected with HIV. I believe, as the CDC does, that the disclosure must occur when procedures are performed which put the patient at risk of exposure.[58]

Exactly what the CDC believed about patient notification was still not clear, unfortunately. While the CDC officials had repeatedly pledged to offer a public comment period on their proposed recommendations, the offer was withdrawn when the final recommendations were actually issued. As CDC director Roper argued, "we believe we've had a very open process with lots of people commenting, and what we need now is to go forward with the guidelines." He added that although "we're very sensitive to the issue since we said we would have

a comment period," the CDC was under no legal obligation to provide one.[59] Furthermore, the agency was already embarrassed that it
had taken as long as it had to develop the guidelines, and it wanted to
avoid the flood of letters certain to follow any call for comments.

It is important to note the magnitude of the last-minute changes
to the guidelines. The difference between *should* notify patients and
would notify them is enormous. *Should* implies an ethical obligation;
would indicates a legal one. Like all CDC guidelines, however, these
provided advice but not commands. As a result, even though the
guidelines now indicated that HIV-positive HCWs needed to notify
patients, the CDC could not compel them to do so.

Congress could. Senators Ted Kennedy (D–Massachusetts) and
Hatch, supported by the leadership of both parties, subsequently
introduced an amendment (to the same appropriations bill), requiring
"states to adopt the recommendations of the CDC concerning the
transmission of the HIV virus by [health care workers] to patients."[60]
(This controversy had not caught Kennedy and Hatch entirely by surprise. On October 11, 1990, shortly after the CDC's first consultants
meeting, Roper had written a letter to both senators alerting them to
the fact that the CDC was reviewing its guidelines for HIV-infected
health care workers.) States that did not adopt these recommendations, or equivalent ones, would not be eligible to receive funding
assistance from the Public Health Service. This amendment was
offered in the hope that the Senate would adopt it instead of the
Helms amendment. This hope was not met. The Kennedy-Hatch
amendment did pass unanimously (ninety-nine to zero). But the Senate also enacted the Helms amendment by an overwhelming vote
(eighty-one to eighteen). In explaining these votes, Senator Peter
DeConcini noted that they gave "political cover where [senators]
couldn't be criticized for being too tough or too soft."[61] It was also a
"free" vote; because the House was not considering similar legislation,
the senators knew that the Helms amendment would not become
law.[62] The senators could vote for a popular idea without having to
worry that the vote would actually affect policy.

Now it was the House's turn. Rather than slipping amendments
into an appropriations bill—which House rules forbid—the House
Subcommittee on Health and the Environment made a public display
of its concerns by holding hearings on Dannemeyer's Kimberly
Bergalis Act as promised.[63] The highlight was to be, of course, Kimberly's own testimony. But in the days before she appeared, a broad

range of views, often echoing those heard at the CDC's open meetings, was presented. While congressional hearings are often designed with drama in mind—advocates and opponents of legislative proposals are inclined to invite the most sensational witnesses—they can also provide a public forum for serious consideration of the issues.

Chair Waxman began the hearings by stating that "we must focus on the known risks and true responses, not on the feared risks or easy responses. The quick answer is often not the right one. We should protect the public health, always. . . . And that protection should be urgent, calm, and compassionate."[64] Dannemeyer, in his opening comments, argued in contrast that the "the CDC has developed a computer model that tells us today that there are 128 Kimberly Bergalises in this country. . . . There has been a failure of leadership on the part of public health authorities . . . [who] treat this as a civil rights issue, that somehow the civil rights of the infected take precedence over the civil rights of the uninfected."[65]

One of the first speakers was former surgeon general C. Everett Koop. Koop, a Reagan appointee, had made a name for himself by challenging social conservatives on several issues in sexuality, including abortion and sexual education, and he was no more a captive of the conservatives on this issue than he was on any other. Koop argued that the risk of being infected with HIV by a health care worker "is so remote that it may never be measured." Requiring all health care workers to be tested would thus be "worthless."[66] Koop's comments were seconded by numerous medical groups (such as the American Medical Association, the American College of Emergency Physicians, the American Nurses Association, and the American Dental Association) as well as the CDC.

Bergalis arrived in Washington by train on September 25. She was the first of fifteen witnesses to testify the next day. Her testimony lasted just seconds: "AIDS is a terrible disease that you must take seriously. I did nothing wrong, yet I'm being made to suffer like this. My life has been taken away. Please enact legislation so no other patient and health care provider will have to go through the hell that I have. Thank you."[67]

Her father, testifying next, spoke more bluntly to the members of Congress: "Kimberly is your shame. . . . She is a result of your unwillingness or inability to deal with this [AIDS] monster you created. . . . One day we all will be held accountable by our ultimate judge. We will face that day with a clear conscience. Will you?"[68]

Afterward, the Bergalis family joined in a press conference featuring both proponents and opponents of the bill. Her parents were irate:

> Our daughter literally got off her deathbed to come here and testify. She isn't looking for emotion. She isn't looking for sorrow. She came here to make a passionate plea today for a bill to require AIDS testing of health care workers.
>
> Dr. Acer might as well have shot her in the head. He caused her to die. Her dying wish, which maybe this is, is that members of Congress cast their vote on this.
>
> The health care bureaucracy cares more for their income and their own rights than they do for their patients' health. When this country has decided that someone's civil rights, their ability to earn a living, is more important than someone's life, it is time to make a change.[69]

> I'm frustrated with people who say that mandatory testing of medical workers would not be effective—that it's unnecessary and would cost too much. I get tested every year for tuberculosis, and if I have TB, I can't practice [as a nurse]. Dr. Acer practiced four years with AIDS.
>
> I think it's ironic that what was probably our daughter's last trip was here to Washington. Where did my daughter's AIDS originate? Here, with uncaring politicians.[70]

When persons such as David Rogers, vice chair of the National AIDS Commission, spoke out against mandatory testing at this press conference ("the overwhelming scientific evidence tells us the testing of health care [professionals] is not going to contribute much to reducing transmission of AIDS"), the Bergalises objected, "Why can't they see how important this is? Bureaucrats!"[71]

The same day, back in Florida, one of these bureaucrats was also speaking out. Unlike the Bergalis testimony and press conference, which were covered by all the major media, his comments were carried deep inside a single local newspaper. But Florida's top AIDS administrator, John Witte, was a rare public official to speak out against what Bergalis was doing:

> The Kimberly Bergalis episode has created an enormous amount of hysteria and anxiety among the general public. . . . Of course, what she's going to say is that we need mandatory testing. . . . [But her

testimony] is adding to the fear, and we need to make decisions based on scientific data, not fear of the unknown.[72]

A spokesman for the state AIDS program went on to say that biannual HIV tests for Florida HCWs would cost $50 million, virtually bankrupting the already overextended state health care budget.

The House resisted Helms's intemperate call to throw HIV-infected health care workers in prison as well as Bergalis's plea for mandatory testing. Indeed, no votes were taken on the Bergalis Act, and it died in committee. When the House-Senate conference committee began to resolve the differences between their respective versions of the legislation, it quietly dropped Helms's punishments on individuals.[73] The House negotiators, for their part, were less than enthusiastic about the Kennedy-Hatch proposals. House Democrats objected, in particular, to the idea that the states could lose their entire Public Health Service funding—including money to immunize children—if they failed to adopt the CDC's guidelines. As Representative Nancy Pelosi (D–California) put it, "to go after this problem with a sledgehammer when a feather would do, that's excessive."[74] Yet the Senate negotiators were not willing to reverse direction completely. One staffer noted, "The Senate position was [that] we cannot weaken the language to the point that we drop [the Helms amendment] and then backslide [on the Kennedy-Hatch proposal] too."[75] Ultimately the Senate's version stuck, and so Public Law 102–141 required the states to adopt the CDC guidelines, or else.

Why did Congress take the action that it did? Political scientist William Gormley provides some insight. He argues that when a political issue is highly "salient"—that is, when the public is extremely concerned about it—Congress is much more likely to take action than when an issue is not salient.[76] The Bergalis case was extraordinarily salient, so Congress acted. No surprise there. The insight is that Congress can take action in one of two ways. Just like the CDC with its recommendations, it can enact "substantive" legislation (describing what must be done to solve the problem) or "procedural" legislation (establishing the method for solving the problem). The Helms amendment is an example of the former ("we solve the problem by imprisoning HIV-infected HCWs who continue practicing"); the Kennedy-Hatch proposal exemplifies the latter ("we solve the problem by telling the states to follow the CDC guidelines"). Congress seems to prefer adopting substantive legislation if the policy issue is

technically simple (that is, when it does not require specialized expertise to resolve) and procedural bills when it is technically complex.

The technical complexity of this issue is, admittedly, subject to
debate. In the eyes of the public (and the Helms amendment), the
issue was simple: test health care workers for HIV and do not let the
infected ones provide medical care without notifying their patients.
The Kennedy-Hatch proposal, in contrast, took the view that the decisions regarding health care providers and HIV would best be made by
public health experts (namely, the CDC). While the Senate had mixed
views about which interpretation was appropriate and thus enacted
both, Congress appeared ultimately to be persuaded that the issue was
better handled by experts in public health. Senator Kennedy was
explicit on this point:

> This is the critical issue before us. And the question now to be con-
> sidered by the Senate is whether we believe that the best answer to [the
> problem of HIV-infected health care workers] would be sending some-
> one to prison for ten years . . . and also imposing a $10,000 fine, or
> whether we should take the recommendations of the Centers for Dis-
> ease Control and implement the newly released guidelines. These rec-
> ommendations of the CDC represent the best thinking of our
> scientists and the medical profession, which have been studying and
> reviewing this issue for the last year. This has entailed thousands of
> pages of paper, days of testimony, and hours of consideration, all given
> to this one question: What is going to be the best public health policy
> for this country that will protect our patients and health care profes-
> sionals?[77]

IMPLEMENTATION FAILS

The CDC's recommendations, for all the effort taken to produce them,
did not finally answer this question. The practical meaning of the
CDC's recommendations for the states was far from clear, to put it
mildly. They indicated, for instance, that only those physicians who
performed "exposure-prone" (that is, potentially risky) procedures
needed to learn whether they were infected with HIV (mandatory testing was not recommended), to seek counsel from expert panels
regarding their ability to perform these procedures, and to disclose
their HIV status to their patients. But what *exactly* were these risky
procedures? The CDC did provide some guidance, noting that

"characteristics of exposure-prone procedures include digital palpa-
tion of a needle tip in a body cavity or the simultaneous presence of
the HCW's fingers and a needle or other sharp instrument or object
in a poorly visualized or highly confined anatomic site."[78]

Procedures with these attributes included "certain oral, cardiotho-
racic, colorectal, and obstetric/gynecologic procedures."[79] The CDC
went on to say that "performance of exposure-prone procedures presents a recognized risk of percutaneous [through the skin] injury to
the HCW, and—if such an injury occurs—the HCW's blood is likely
to contact the patient's [bloodstream]." Still, the CDC suggested that
the exact set of procedures should be identified by medical, surgical,
and dental organizations and the institutions where the procedures
are performed.[80] CDC director Roper set November 15, 1991, as the
deadline for these organizations to develop their lists.

This was easier said than done. On November 4, at a meeting it
hosted to discuss the risky procedures, the CDC faced a barrage of
criticism from health care and civil rights groups.[81] "The question we
have to ask ourselves is—is [the idea for identifying a list of risky pro-
cedures] based on scientific merit or an overreactive response to political pressure," said Quentin Stiles of the Society of Thoracic
Surgeons.[82] Neil Schram, from the American Association of Physicians
for Human Rights, gave the answer: "We are here for political reasons.
We are not here for medical reasons."[83] The opposition from the medical, surgical, and dental organizations (among others) was intense.
These groups made several main claims. *No* specific medical procedures had been linked to the accidental transmission of HIV from
physician to patient. As a result, there was *no* empirical basis for concluding that any procedures created greater risks of transmitting HIV
to patients than did any other procedures. The medical groups essentially offered the slogan: "Procedures don't kill people, (incompetent)
providers do." Most providers, it was argued, virtually never exposed
their blood to their patients even when performing quite difficult
operations; other providers perhaps cut themselves doing even easy
procedures. (Remember, Acer had performed routine tooth extractions on Bergalis but simply cleaned Sherry Johnson's teeth.) By the
time the meeting ended, more than thirty organizations—including
the American College of Surgeons, the American College of Physicians, and the American Dental Association—refused to cooperate
with the CDC in drawing up the list of exposure-prone procedures.
Walter Lamacki, speaking for the dentists, argued that the risk of den-

tists infecting patients was "infinitesimal" and stated flatly that the ADA could not provide a list of risky procedures.[84]

Only the American Medical Association continued to agree with the CDC that such a list was necessary and appropriate, arguing in the words of its representative, Nancy Dickey, that it was "simply unacceptable to stand by, wait, and watch for possible cases of health care workers infecting patients with HIV in order to bring more scientific confidence to our recommendations."[85] The AMA was conspicuously silent in making suggestions for the contents of this list, however.[86] Ultimately it, too, refused to identify specific procedures.[87] The revolt must have discouraged the CDC, although Roper put the best face on it: "We are anxious to proceed in a manner that builds consensus," he said. "We are going to think very clearly about this in the next few weeks."[88]

The revolt also left both the CDC and the states in a bind. The CDC was ill prepared either politically or professionally to identify risky medical procedures without the cooperation of the broader medical community. The states, on the other hand, were left to wonder how they could comply with recommendations so nebulous that the CDC itself could not define them.

Concluding that it would be impossible to develop a list of risky procedures and so to require HCWs who performed them to disclose their HIV status to their patients, CDC officials considered revising its recommendations to drop these sections.[89] The revised guidelines were to suggest that professional restrictions should be placed only on those health care workers who posed a "significant risk" to patients that "could not be modified by reasonable accommodations" in accordance with the Americans with Disabilities Act.[90] Efforts to issue new recommendations were soon dropped, however, after the case was made that the proposed changes would violate the will of Congress. As Assistant Secretary Mason argued, "the decision [to drop the proposals] was a legal and statutory one. . . . The legal people felt that any changes in the guidelines had to be examined within the context of the law passed by Congress, and that you couldn't switch the guidelines without going back to [Capitol] Hill."[91]

It was time to punt. Roper sent a letter to all fifty state health departments, telling them their guidelines would be considered "equivalent" to the CDC's if they decided "that exposure-prone invasive procedures are best determined on a case-by-case basis, taking into consideration the specific procedure as well as the skill, technique, and possible impairment of the infected health care worker."[92] As a CDC public affairs officer explained, "what is exposure-prone for one health care worker may not be for another. It's better to have local boards decide on each case."[93] Perhaps it was better, but it certainly was no easier. As the next chapter shows, every organization responsible for resolving the controversies surrounding HIV and HCWs has struggled to find sensible and acceptable answers.

CHAPTER SEVEN

Dilemmas
States, Regulators, and Courts Address the Controversies

T he CDC, under congressional pressure, had
finally produced new guidelines for HCWs and HIV. Congress,
responding to public demands, incorporated these guidelines into law.
The CDC, trying to resolve the meaning of its own recommendations,
then found that it could not. Congress and the CDC thus followed an
American political tradition: they acted when necessary, but in doing
so they passed the tough decisions on to someone else.

So the CDC guidelines and Congress's law were not the end of this
story. In American public policy the cliché "it's not over 'til it's over"
does not apply. A more accurate description would be "it's never over,
even when it's over." In America, no political institution has ultimate
authority, and no policy decisions are final. Our government is so fragmented across federal, state, and local levels, as well as within executive, legislative, and judicial branches at each level, that decisions made
by any governmental actors can be elaborated, implemented, appealed,
or ignored by the others.

THE STATES' RESPONSE

Congress, by requiring the states to adopt guidelines "equivalent" to those of the CDC, gave instructions without much content. The CDC, by instructing the local health boards to decide such critical issues as which procedures were exposure prone, did the same. And the states and local health boards found it no easier to resolve matters concerning HIV-infected health care workers than Congress or the CDC had.

Let us look first at what the states did *not* do. Despite the apparently overwhelming public support for mandatory testing, no state has passed legislation requiring that HCWs be tested for HIV, although bills to do so were introduced in at least six states (Delaware, Florida, Maryland, New Hampshire, South Carolina, and Texas).[1] It is especially notable that these bills failed in Maryland, even though its governor expressed strong support for the bill, and in Florida, home of the Bergalis incident. Maryland's governor, Donald Schaefer, favored testing so strongly that he "scrapped" his AIDS advisory panel, arguing that its members were more concerned about confidentiality than public health.[2] In Florida, state senator John McKay, who introduced a bill requiring HCWs and patients both to be tested, abandoned the legislation after researching its "fiscal feasibility."[3]

A few states did define certain situations in which patients may request or compel health care providers to be tested for HIV. Virginia law, for instance, specifies that a provider who directly exposes a patient to the provider's bodily fluids (as defined by the CDC) will be deemed to have consented to HIV testing and the release of the test results to the exposed patient; West Virginia and Oregon have similar laws. Notably, these laws were all passed prior to the Florida dentist case.[4] In the absence of additional administrative guidance, individual HCWs in all states, in almost all situations, will continue to determine if, when, and how often they will be tested. At least in terms of testing, Bergalis's wishes have not prevailed in the states; the experts' view has.[5]

The issue of patient notification has been even more contentious and the results less clear. The states, if they are to have policies equivalent to the CDC's, must require HIV-infected health care providers to disclose this fact to their patients before performing exposure-prone procedures on them. But in fact, this has not happened even in those states, such as Texas, that adopted the CDC recommendations verbatim and so by law require patient notification. Because the CDC was never able to define "exposure-prone" procedures, this component of the law has had little or no practical impact. It appears that no states are enforcing any requirements that HIV-positive HCWs routinely disclose their diagnosis to their patients before treating them.

At least some states are struggling with the issue, however. Consider the situation in New York, which had faced controversies involving HIV-positive HCWs before the Bergalis case was announced.[6] In a prominent legal case, a pharmacist was denied employment by a hospital based on the "risk to patients" he presumably posed by preparing intravenous pharmaceuticals.[7] Even though the infectious disease control director of the hospital argued that the pharmacist presented negligible risk to the patients, the hospital justified its decision not to hire him by referring to the CDC's 1987 recommendations that all infected HCWs should be subject to individual review.[8] It took seventeen expert witnesses and a year of trial for the state to conclude that the pharmacist should not be restricted in his duties.

At that point the New York state legislature directed the state Department of Health to define exactly what "significant risk" meant as it pertained to health care workers and HIV.[9] According to the Health Department, HCWs who used "scientifically accepted barrier techniques and preventive practices" did *not* pose significant risks. As a result, HIV-infected HCWs should not be restricted—even from invasive procedures—as long as they were competent in infection control practices, if they had not been linked to any infective incidents, and if they were otherwise functionally able to continue employment.[10] In January 1991, months before the CDC issued its new guidelines, the New York Health Department adopted its comprehensive policy for HIV-infected HCWs, which reiterated that these persons should not have their practices restricted unless they had functional impairments or lacked competence in infection control. The New York guidelines, moreover, explicitly allowed infected HCWs to perform invasive procedures without revealing their HIV status to their patients so long as the provider followed universal precautions.[11] Indeed, New York state health officials rejected the CDC's guidelines when they were finally issued.[12] Massachusetts immediately followed suit, and Michigan also rejected compulsory disclosure.[13]

The New York guidelines were almost immediately questioned, however, by the New York State Supreme Court (which despite its name is not the highest court of appeals in New York) in a case involving a New York dentist who died from AIDS.[14] After Dr. Feldman's death, it was widely reported in the local press that he had a substance abuse problem and that he did not follow universal precautions in treating patients. The state publicly offered to provide HIV tests for Feldman's patients, but only 650 of his approximately 3,000 patients accepted the offer. In order to contact personally the other patients, the state Health Department sued to obtain Feldman's patient records. The court ruled in favor of the department but noted with some irony that the department did not require providers to disclose their HIV status *before* they treated patients, although it did attempt to inform the patients *after* they received treatment. The court spoke strongly in favor of patients' rights to know the HIV status of their health care providers, while noting that if public health authorities chose to limit this right, they should at least identify HIV-positive providers so that they could be carefully monitored to ensure that they did not pose risks to patient health. Legislation was subsequently introduced into New York that would have imposed criminal sanctions against providers who are HIV infected and did not obtain informed consent from their patients before treating them. This measure did not pass, nor did any of the bills in six other states that would have provided criminal sanctions against HIV-infected health care workers.[15]

In some states, the law does call for patients to be notified if it can be determined that the provider may have already exposed the patient to HIV.[16] In Illinois, for example, the law directs the state Health Department to determine whether each reported case of AIDS presents a possible risk of HIV transmission.[17] Any HCW who has AIDS and performs "invasive procedures" (as defined by the CDC) would be considered to present such a risk. The patients, accordingly, would be notified that they had had a potential exposure to HIV. Still, the HCW would not need to notify the patient in advance nor would the HCW's identity be revealed to the patient afterward.

The states have thus done no better job than the federal government in specifying the conditions under which HCWs must disclose their HIV status to patients. State laws generally accept the concept that only HCWs performing exposure-prone procedures could potentially transmit HIV to patients, but they do not define what these procedures are. Like the federal government, state legislation delegates the definition of "exposure prone" to medical authorities. Medical authorities in the states, however, are no closer to defining these procedures specifically than when the CDC issued its guidelines.

Following the CDC, most states have delegated to various medical groups the power to make decisions regarding which HIV-positive HCWs may continue what practices under which circumstances. A few states have specified some conditions that preclude HCWs from practicing. Missouri and Texas, for example, have prohibited providers with exposed lesions or "weeping dermatitis" from performing certain procedures. No medical panel would have allowed HCWs to provide patient treatment in these circumstances, however, so the benefit of these laws is unclear. As a result, state legislation appears to have taken an uncontroversial middle ground between what patients wanted and what experts preferred by making some easy decisions about the restrictions of HCWs' practices while leaving the tough calls to others such as the health care workers and their employers.

Yet other states chose to focus on universal precautions. At least six states (California, Iowa, Maryland, Minnesota, Missouri, and Oklahoma) have enacted laws specifically requiring health care providers to use universal precautions and imposing sanctions on those who do not.[18] These sanctions typically involve revocation or suspension of license rather than criminal penalties. At least five other states (Delaware, Florida, New York, South Carolina, and Virginia) have also enacted legislation mandating that certain providers receive training in universal precautions as part of their instructional requirements.[19] The laws do not spell out how universal precautions will be monitored, and it is doubtful that the states are expending many of their health care resources on monitoring.

States apparently are spending a fair amount to educate and train health care workers about HIV and AIDS, however. An AIDS Policy Center survey in 1992 showed that only four states (Arkansas, Minnesota, New Mexico, and Texas) were not conducting statewide educational programs; thirty-nine states reported spending almost $16 million in state and federal funds in these programs. California, Florida, Michigan, New York, and Virginia each spent over $1 million.[20] Interestingly, the provisions mandating universal precautions link the goals of patients and experts, as the policies recognize that infection control is a key to preventing HIV transmission (the expert view) and that health care providers must be compelled to use them to reduce the risk (the patient intent).

By 1993, fifteen states had enacted some form of law for HIV-positive health care workers, with at least eight states adopting some form of the CDC guidelines or their equivalent. Twenty-one states had enacted legislation requiring HCWs to take education and training courses in universal precautions, HIV prevention, or both.[21] Many states had taken administrative action to comply with the CDC guidelines. Still, "delay" was the most popular form of compliance with the law requiring states to adopt policies equivalent to the CDC guidelines; in 1992, twenty states were granted their requests for extensions to develop their own HIV policies. For the states, at least this much was certain: they were not eager to lose their Public Health Service (PHS) funding (nor was the CDC enthused about stripping it from them). All fifty states, the District of Columbia, and six territories received their PHS funds in 1993 and every year since, because the CDC approved their efforts to comply with the congressional mandate. For now, all the states have policies equivalent to the CDC's guidelines, whatever that means.

ENTER THE REGULATORS

In 1986, three years before Kimberly Bergalis first visited David Acer, the U.S. Occupational Safety and Health Administration (OSHA) was beginning to formulate new rules regarding bloodborne pathogens such as HIV and hepatitis.[22] This was not the first time; already in 1983 OSHA had issued voluntary guidelines to reduce the risk of occupational exposure to the hepatitis B virus for employees in health care facilities. In September 1986, several large labor unions (including the American Federation of State, County, and Municipal Employees and the Service Employees International Union) began to seek regulatory protection for their members who were routinely exposed to blood through their jobs. Then, in May 1987, the CDC announced the first cases of HIV among health care workers with no documented risk factors other than occupational exposure to the virus.[23] Later that same month, Senator Ted Kennedy introduced legislation (the AIDS Research and Information Act) directing the secretary of HHS to develop guidelines for preventing transmission of HIV and hepatitis to health care and public safety workers (patients were not mentioned) and then to transmit these guidelines to the secretary of labor to be used by OSHA in developing its standards.[24]

OSHA had been created in 1970 "to assure, so far as possible, safe and healthful working conditions for every American worker over the period of his or her working lifetime."[25] OSHA was given authority to develop regulations and to enforce them through inspecting work-places and fining violators. The Supreme Court has ruled, however, that before OSHA can develop regulations, the agency has to make two findings.[26] First, it must demonstrate that a place of employment is unsafe because it has "significant risks." Second, it has to show that these risks could be reduced by a change in practices. Once OSHA has determined that a significant risk exists and could be reduced, it is empowered to set regulatory standards "which most adequately assure, to the extent feasible, on the basis of the best available evidence, that no employee will suffer material impairment of health or functional capacity even if such employee has regular exposure to the hazard dealt with by such standard for the period of his working life."[27]

The Supreme Court has interpreted this to mean that OSHA must enact the most protective standard possible to eliminate a significant risk of material health impairment, subject to the constraints of tech-nological and economic feasibility.[28] The Court did not specify exactly when OSHA must act, however; instead, it said that "scientific cer-tainty" need not exist for risks to be identified, that no "mathematical straitjacket" should be used to determine which risks were significant, and that the significance of risk would largely be based on "policy con-siderations."[29]

Senator Kennedy's request that OSHA develop standards to pro-tect health care workers was certainly one such policy consideration. In response, OSHA at first seemed to leap into action—at least compared to OSHA's normally sluggish pace. By the end of October 1987, OSHA and the CDC (through the Department of Labor and HHS, their respective departments) wrote and sent a "Joint Advisory Notice" regarding HIV and hepatitis in the health care setting to some six hun-dred thousand employers, employee representatives, and trade and professional associations urging the "widest possible adherence to the CDC guidelines and [this] notice." OSHA also used its existing pow-ers to enforce these guidelines; during the next six months, OSHA would inspect fifty-nine health care facilities and issue nine citations.[30]

OSHA followed up by posting its "Advance Notice of Proposed Regulations" in the *Federal Register* on November 27, 1987. (OSHA, unlike the CDC, was bound by the Administrative Procedures Act.) This notice solicited comments from the public regarding the scope and content of the rules. In the mild words of OSHA, its advanced notice received "an overwhelming response."[31] While OSHA was trying to sort out these responses, Kennedy's AIDS Research and

Information Act became law in April 1988, and that same month Kennedy held oversight hearings on OSHA, pressing it for a commitment on the standards. Then, in June 1988, the CDC released its new universal precaution guidelines—the set prevailing during the Florida dentist case.

It took OSHA almost eighteen months, from November 1987 until May 1989, to digest the comments it received, develop its proposed regulations, and publish them in the *Federal Register*.[32] During the fall of that year, OSHA held public hearings on the proposed rule in Washington, D.C., Chicago, New York, Miami, and San Francisco—the cities in which the most health care workers were likely to be exposed to HIV. At these hearings, over four hundred people, representing the wide range of interested parties, including health care providers, labor unions, trade and professional organizations, and other affected parties, testified. The public comment period on the proposed regulations, which ended on May 21, 1990, contained 4,500 separate entries, making it "the largest substantive record in agency history." Undaunted by the volume of responses, OSHA officials testifying before Congress promised that the agency intended to give "careful consideration" to every comment.[33]

This was not the only promise OSHA was to give, as OSHA pledged to issue its final rules first within a year, then by September 1991, and then by the spring of 1992.[34] It missed each self-imposed deadline. (To be sure, not all the delay should be attributed to OSHA. Proposed regulations had to be cleared by the Office of Management and Budget before they could be published. And, during the Reagan and Bush administrations, OMB had imposed lengthy delays on the regulatory efforts of the agencies.) Five full years after it began developing regulations for bloodborne pathogens—making the CDC appear almost reckless in its speed—OSHA still had not issued final rules.

As with the CDC, Congress then attempted to force the action. The Senate leadership, both Democrat and Republican, proposed legislation that required OSHA to announce final rules by December 1, 1991. If OSHA were unable to do this, the standards OSHA had proposed on May 30, 1989—based on the recommendations of the CDC—would go into effect.[35]

Much of the testimony reported in the *Congressional Record* at this time regarding the need for a rule involved the Bergalis case. Former surgeon general Everett Koop, speaking on behalf of OSHA's proposed rule, devoted almost his entire speech to the Bergalis case, noting in particular the public fear of contracting HIV from HCWs even though Acer's patients were the only ones to be infected in this way out of the 187,000 Americans who by then had developed AIDS.[36] Senator Alan Cranston went so far as to claim, with dubious accuracy, that "if the OSHA bloodborne standard had been in place and enforced, the suspected transmission of HIV infection to Kimberly Bergalis and four other patients of a Florida dentist would likely not have occurred."[37]

Under congressional pressure, OSHA finally issued its 178-page "Occupational Exposure to Bloodborne Pathogens" rule on December 6, 1991.[38] These standards were designed to require all employers to ensure that their employees used universal precautions. They were expected to cover 5.6 million workers (including 4.5 million health care employees) who are "reasonably anticipated" to come into contact with blood on the job and, as a beneficial side effect, to protect all patients against exposure to bloodborne diseases. (The standard covers not only workers employed in hospitals, physicians' and dentists' offices, research laboratories, and nursing homes but also employees of many other facilities. These include correctional institutions, law enforcement agencies, and emergency response agencies, as well as institutions for the developmentally disabled, funeral homes, linen services, handlers of infectious wastes, and medical equipment service and repair companies. Medical, nursing, dental, and allied health students are not included under the OSHA standard unless they happen also to be employees. Employees of state, county, or municipal facilities are generally exempt, as OSHA does not directly regulate them. Twenty-five states, however, have state OSHA programs that have been approved by the federal OSHA, so employees in these states are covered.) While consistent with the CDC guidelines on universal precautions, one main difference is that the OSHA standard has an enforcement mechanism to help ensure that these precautions are followed.

The OSHA standard used the full range of its available tools in essentially adopting the portion of the CDC guidelines regarding infection control. Employers, including physicians, have to develop a written exposure control plan that identifies tasks, procedures, and job classifications involving exposure to infectious materials. A "methods of compliance" section mandates the use of universal precautions and describes in detail what these precautions are. The rule requires that all employers train their employees regarding the OSHA standards. (In addition, vaccination for hepatitis has to be offered free, with easy access, and under specified medical supervision to all occupational exposure-prone employees within ten workdays of their assignment. Employees can choose not to be vaccinated, however.) Strict and sometimes onerous record-keeping rules are imposed; for example, employers are required to keep detailed confidential medical records for the duration of employment plus *thirty years* for any employee with occupational exposure to HIV or hepatitis. Employers who are not in compliance with the rules can be fined based on the seriousness of the violation. Citations for serious violations can result in penalties of up to $7,000 per violation per day; willful or repeated violations of the standard can be fined up to $70,000 for each violation.

Despite taking five years to develop the rule, considering thousands of pages of comments, and hearing hundreds of hours of testimony, OSHA was nonetheless sued for its regulations. (Actually, OSHA is sued over virtually every major regulation it issues.[39]) The American Dental Association (ADA) and the Home Health Services and Staffing Association (HHSSA), supported by the American College of Surgeons (ACS), sought to have a moratorium imposed on the regulations.[40]

Their challenge was based on four grounds. First, they claimed that OSHA failed to establish that a significant risk existed within dental clinics and among home health providers and thus that it had no basis for regulating them. Second, they argued that OSHA failed to establish that the final rule would result in substantial benefit to these health care workers, especially given that the CDC and the states were already taking actions to prevent infections. Third (as a touch of public relations?), ADA and HHSSA maintained that the rule was aimed only at protecting employees and thus lacked concern for and failed to protect the consumer (that is, patients) because it increased health care costs and at the same time denied patients access to essential information (such as the HCW's HIV status) necessary to the granting of informed consent. Finally, the plaintiffs maintained that there were flaws in OSHA's feasibility analysis.

The federal Seventh Circuit Court rejected these claims in January 1993. But like everything else involving HIV and health care workers, there was no unanimity of opinion, as the court decided by a two-to-one majority to allow OSHA to implement its rule. Judge Posner, while offering some criticisms of OSHA and its rule and finding some merit in ADA's position, nonetheless found that

OSHA's evaluation of the effects of the rule, relying as it does on the undoubted expertise of the Centers for Disease Control, cannot seriously be faulted, at least by judges. Hence we cannot say that the rule, viewed as a whole, flunks the test of material reduction of a significant risk to workplace health.[41]

In particular, Judge Posner noted that in developing its regulations, OSHA did not—in fact, was not permitted to—consider whether its rules would pass a cost-benefit analysis. By law, OSHA is instructed only to consider whether its rules would "materially reduce a significant workplace risk to human health without imperiling the existence of, or threatening massive dislocation to, the health care industry."[42] In Posner's opinion, OSHA's regulations passed both these tests.

As far as reducing workplace risks, OSHA had estimated that each year the rule would save almost 300 lives. Only a handful of lives were expected to be saved by preventing HIV transmission, however; almost all would be saved by preventing the spread of hepatitis. OSHA estimated that the rule would result in between 113 and 129 fewer health care workers infected with hepatitis each year and that, as a side benefit, these workers in turn would not infect between 187 and 197 patients. OSHA also estimated that its rules would prevent about 9,200 other cases of bloodborne infection each year.[43]

In making these estimates, OSHA also guessed that compliance would cost $813 million each year, which in Posner's view was "clearly not enough to break the multi-hundred-billion-dollar health care industry."[44] (OSHA estimated that the rule would cost dentistry less than one-third of 1 percent of the industry's annual revenues. The Court noted that these costs were almost certainly underestimated because they did not accurately reflect the time and effort spent on complying with them.) Implicitly, then, OSHA expected that it would cost about $4 million to save each life. By regulatory standards, this was a high but hardly unprecedented value placed on saving lives.[45] Because HIV and hepatitis often kill persons relatively early in their lives and because these diseases cause much misery before death, they are considered "costly" diseases.

Still, Posner also noted that some lives might be lost as a consequence of the rule and that OSHA did not attempt to estimate these losses. How could the rule cost lives? The logic goes like this: the rule raises overall health care costs, and these costs will be passed on to consumers. As the price of health care rises, the demand for health care will fall; fewer services will be provided. The reduction in services would potentially endanger some persons' health.[46]

Judge Coffey, in his dissenting opinion, argued that the dentists and home health care workers were mainly correct on every point.[47] OSHA's "fatal error," Coffey argued, was that it did not consider the varying risks of occupational exposure to HIV and hepatitis experienced by different health care workers or that most dental and home health care professionals essentially had zero risk of being infected (or infecting others).[48]

Indeed, at the time that OSHA developed the rule, only a single dental worker had been identified as having contracted HIV through providing care, and apparently no home health care workers had been so infected. It was not crystal clear, moreover, that this one dentist had contracted HIV from a patient. The dentist did not know whether he had treated patients with AIDS, although he reported that he treated patients at "high risk" of being infected. He reported having frequent open lesions or "obvious breaks in the skin" on his hands and intermittently using personal protective equipment. The dentist denied having any other risk factors, as did his wife (who refused to be tested for HIV). The uncertainties in this case are that it was not known when the dentist became infected or whether he treated patients with HIV.[49] Judge Coffey thus concluded that:

> The [OSHA] rule adopted can best be classified as an attempt to try to kill a fly with a sledgehammer. The rule was drafted partially in response to the public hysteria surrounding AIDS created by the media's failure to balance their reporting with scientific data on transmission. The rule was not drafted in response to an established significant risk of harm to employees. . . . Based on the record, I am forced to assume that because of the excessive media coverage regarding the AIDS virus, fueled by one single episode involving Kimberly Bergalis in Florida contracting AIDS from her dentist, OSHA decided to promulgate this over-expansive rule . . . [that] unduly burdens health care employers, including but not limited to dentists, doctors, and hospitals, while offering but minimal benefit to their employees.[50]

Coffey also noted that it had been reported that Acer may have intentionally infected his patients. If this was true, Coffey argued, then "no amount of precaution could have prevented it." Still, Coffey was sympathetic to the concerns of patients. In Coffey's view, the root of much of this dispute was a vocal minority's emphasis on the rights of the individual at the expense of the common good of all.

> The defeat of the congressional attempt to require mandatory testing of health care workers can only be explained by powerful lobbying efforts. It is incumbent upon Congress to address . . . the AIDS problem and achieve a balance that reflects the paramount interest of all mankind and not let the overriding concern be with the individual's right of privacy.[51]

With regard to flies and sledgehammers, however, the mandatory HIV testing that the judge apparently favored would (arguably) save fewer lives at greater cost while violating rights of patients and HCWs than the OSHA rule of which Coffey was so critical. The "powerful lobbying efforts" of those who opposed mandatory testing consisted largely of pointing this out.

In one interesting twist, Judge Coffey noted that the Supreme Court had ruled that OSHA regulations preempted any comparable state rules.[52] Because Congress had required the states to adopt rules equivalent to the CDC's guidelines, each state presumably had (or would have) such regulations. As a result, OSHA's regulations effectively trumped CDC's guidelines. Nonetheless, Judge Coffey wondered whether OSHA was competent to regulate the health care workplace or whether Congress had intended OSHA to regulate it. Noting the CDC's expertise in public health, Coffey speculated as to whether Congress should give the CDC the same inspection and enforcement powers as OSHA. The irony of this position is that the CDC had not been able to develop workable standards, nor did it advocate mandatory testing.

THE COURTS EQUIVOCATE

The lawsuit against OSHA hardly exhausted the possibilities for litigation involving HIV, HCWs, patients, and employers. Surveys show that most persons confronted with a wrongful act, including medical malpractice, do not sue or raise legal defenses.[53] Still, in America there is a tendency to seek to resolve political and policy disputes by turning to the courts, and this tendency has continued with issues related to HIV.[54] But resolutions are difficult to obtain. The courts have addressed the controversies in ways that are ambiguous, inconsistent, or apparently irrational.[55]

Kimberly Bergalis (joined later by Barbara Webb and Richard Driskill) sued, of course. With Robert Montgomery (of the West Palm Beach firm of Montgomery and Larmoyeux) as her attorney, Bergalis filed suit in August 1990 against Acer's insurer, Continental National America Group (CNA) and CIGNA Dental Health of Florida, the health insurer that had referred her to him.

This suit hastened the day the world learned that Kimberly Bergalis was the person mentioned in the *MMWR* as the patient apparently infected with HIV by a dentist. To avoid publicity, her case was filed by Montgomery and Larmoyeux in Palm Beach County as *K. B. v. D. A.* The local press, in its routine screening of court filings, found the case. As word about the case spread, Montgomery's law office was swamped with calls to find out who K. B. was (the media had promptly identified Acer as D. A.). It was at this point that the Bergalis family decided to call a press conference to announce that Kimberly was the one. The Bergalis family did not skimp on legal counsel. Montgomery was a member of the Inner Circle of Advocates, a by-invitation club of the nation's top personal injury lawyers. Prior to representing Bergalis he had already had won twenty jury trials in which his clients had been awarded $1 million or more.

Bergalis (through Montgomery) claimed that Acer had an absolute duty to inform his patients about his condition. As a Florida court of appeals had already ruled in another case in which a physician had misdiagnosed a case of tuberculosis in a patient, who then infected his child, "it is recognized that once a contagious disease is known to exist, a duty arises on the part of the physician to use reasonable care to advise and warn members of the patient's immediate family of the existence and dangers of the disease."[56]

Bergalis consequently alleged that CIGNA was guilty of "vicarious liability, corporate negligence, and negligent misrepresentation." According to the suit, CIGNA had approved dentists and "represented them to be . . . competent to practice dentistry in all respects."[57] The vicarious-liability complaint was based on the idea that CIGNA had "absolute control" over Acer's dental practice, from billing, to referrals, and even to what germicide would be used in the clinic.[58] The corporate negligence claim was founded on the principle that CIGNA was responsible for maintaining quality control and so had a duty to investigate the competence of its health care providers.[59] According to Montgomery, this understanding of corporate negligence stemmed from *Insinga* v. *LaBella,* in which a wrongful death suit was brought against a hospital for allowing a person who masqueraded as a physician to treat patients.[60] He argued that another case, *Harrell* v. *Total Health Care, Inc.,* established the duty of an HMO to provide competent physicians for its subscribers.[61] Finally, Bergalis accused CIGNA of negligent misrepresentation based on its brochures, which proclaimed the professionalism of its providers and the high quality of care its clients would receive.

CNA almost immediately settled the claims for $1 million each to Bergalis, Webb, and Driskill.[62] (Subsequently, CNA became one of the first insurance companies to offer HIV disability coverage for HCWs as an incentive for them to restrict their practices or retire.) CIGNA did not settle. Instead, CIGNA tried to divert the case, to delay the trial, and to discredit the patients' claims. It attempted initially to have the case moved to federal court, arguing that the federal government had preempted all issues relating to HIV and AIDS and thus that federal courts had sole jurisdiction. The federal district court denied this petition and sent the case back to the state courts. Then, in March 1991, CIGNA argued that it needed another year to have the blood of Acer and Bergalis independently sequenced. In response, Bergalis's lawyers requested an expedited trial because of her failing health. The court, sensitive to Bergalis's condition, scheduled the trial to begin by mid August.

At the same time, CIGNA sought to portray Bergalis as having put herself at risk of contracting HIV through her own sexual behavior. At CIGNA's request, Bergalis was examined by Phyllis B. Toon, a gynecologist, in the presence of John Pauley, a gynecologist hired by Montgomery. Toon reported that "patient physical exam compatible with prior intercourse. . . . Exam compatible with HPV [human papilloma virus, often called genital warts, a venereal disease]. . . . Patient commented to me that vaginal exams cannot prove prior sexual activity."[63]

This news, together with Bergalis's videotaped deposition in which she acknowledged having some sexual contact with a boyfriend, was widely publicized after her death. In this, the media's financial interest in satisfying the popular thirst for scandal accorded with CIGNA's hopes for raising doubts concerning Bergalis's claims about the source of her infection.

While CIGNA was trying to discredit Bergalis's account, it was also attempting to poke holes in the scientific evidence linking Acer to her. To this end CIGNA hired Lionel Resnick, chief of the Department of Retrovirology and Research at the Mount Sinai Medical Center in Miami, and Stanley Weiss, director of the Division of Infectious Disease Epidemiology at the University of Medicine and Dentistry of New Jersey, to scrutinize the genetic sequencing work done by Gerald Myers for the CDC.

CIGNA's efforts to discredit Bergalis (and hence the CDC's investigation) were unsuccessful. Bergalis's legal team produced medical evidence indicating that physical exams could not demonstrate whether intercourse had occurred and that Kimberly's condition, at any rate, suggested that it had not; that HPV could be contracted without sexual contact and that, moreover, she had not contracted it. Myers, meanwhile, scrutinized the scrutiny performed by Resnick and Weiss (among others) and submitted a critique to the lawyers arguing that its analysis was riddled with errors.[64] By the end of the first week in April, CIGNA entered into a confidential out-of-court settlement with the Bergalis family for an undisclosed sum. Soon after that, CIGNA also settled with Barbara Webb.

CIGNA did not settle so quickly with Driskill, however. The company argued that Driskill's own sexual behavior and drug use made it likely that he had not contracted HIV from Acer. As with Bergalis, CIGNA's lawyers conducted their own inquiry into Driskill's personal life, and they found persons willing to testify that Driskill had sex with AIDS-infected prostitutes and men. Even Montgomery, his lawyer, admitted that Driskill "had affairs with everything that walked."[65]

Even more so than with Bergalis and Webb, then, the genetic evidence linking Driskill to Acer was critical for establishing that the dentist was the source of the infection. And while the jury in the courtroom ultimately would determine whether CIGNA or Driskill had more convincing evidence, both sides sought to influence the broader court of scientific opinion. Accordingly, Resnick and Weiss, together with several scientists not hired by CIGNA, submitted a paper to the prestigious journal *Science*. (The nondefense scientists included Lawrence Abele, dean of arts and sciences at Florida State University, whose research focused on molecular evolution, and Ronald W. DeBry, Department of Biological Science, Florida State. DeBry and Abele vigorously asserted that they participated in this research as scholars, not expert witnesses for the defense.[66]) Myers and others did the same. Not surprisingly, these papers came to different conclusions. The papers themselves became enmeshed in legal controversies. While the papers were under review by *Science,* circuit judge Robert R. Makemsom ruled that the Weiss and Resnick paper must be turned over to Driskill's lawyers. Because Myers was not working on Driskill's behalf, however, the judge could not force this paper to be turned over to CIGNA. Makemsom then ordered that both documents be sealed— that is, not released to the public at large—so that *Science*'s normal peer review process would not be interrupted. (Weiss and Resnick, by the way, had obtained the genetic data through a Freedom of Information Act request. Because Myers's paper had not yet been published in peer-reviewed journals, at least some observers worried that a chilling effect on federally supported research would occur if scholars had to share their data with others prior to publication.[67])

None of the scientists claimed to prove whether Acer had or had not infected his patients. Resnick and Weiss did not have to show that Acer was "innocent" of infecting Driskill but only that he was not guilty beyond a reasonable doubt. That is exactly what they tried to do, as their essay concluded that "our analyses show that the available data are consistent with both the dental transmission hypothesis and the null hypothesis [that is, that Acer did not infect the patients] and do not yet distinguish between the two."[68] The paper by the CDC's researchers, in contrast, did not claim for a fact that Acer had infected Driskill. Instead, it concluded that "the evidence strongly suggests that Acer was the proximal source for each of the [five patients'] infections."[69] In the court of science, the CDC's case prevailed. Its article was published by *Science* in May 1992, and since then, a couple of articles by other researchers have also supported Myers's conclusions.[70] The paper by Resnick and Weiss was rejected, although it did ultimately appear as a less influential "letter" (that is, a piece not subject to peer review) in *Nature.*[71] Barr, who argued that Acer had not infected his patients, reported (as evidence) that Resnick continued to claim that he planned to submit new research on this case for publication.[72] This research has apparently never been published.

CIGNA, again, was persuaded to settle with Driskill for an undisclosed sum (he had asked for $15 million). Indeed, none of the lawsuits filed by the six patients would ever go to court. Sherry Johnson, settled for "a bunch of money" in January 1994, according to her lawyer Montgomery.[73] Shortly before his death in 1993, Yecs received $50,000 from the rehab program that had referred him to Acer. Shoemaker, it appears, was the odd one out. She had not been referred to Acer by CIGNA, so could not sue it. She did sue CNA, but its policy on Acer had been exhausted by Bergalis, Webb, and Driskill.

These lawsuits provided substantial sums of money, at least to Bergalis, Webb, Driskill, and Johnson. What they did not do, however, is resolve any of the legal or policy questions. After all, defendants in legal cases can reach out-of-court settlements for a wide variety of reasons that have little to do with the merits of the case. It should not be surprising that CIGNA believed it had little chance to win the jury trials; it can be tempting for jurors, seeing the suffering of the patients, to stick it to an impersonal corporation. It would not be astonishing if the patients were also unwilling to face a jury, as it is unpleasant at best to have one's intimate life bared for peers to judge. Cases that go to juries are almost always a big gamble for both sides. But because no court ruled in these cases, no legal precedents were set. Still, these were apparently the first cases in which patients have sued a prepaid dental insurer for the acts of one of its providers and collected substantial sums.

The CDC, which could not prevent all infections, could hardly be expected to prevent all lawsuits. Still, the guidelines it issued in response to the Bergalis case did little to clarify legal matters. Indeed, the guidelines have been blamed for making the legal issues even murkier than they were before.[74] Some patients, even though they had not contracted HIV, nevertheless sued their HIV-infected physicians for "putting them at risk," as the guidelines implied that at least some procedures were risky. In other cases, HIV-positive HCWs sued their employers for relieving them of their duties, claiming that they posed no risk to patients because they did not perform the (undefined) risky procedures. In short, the CDC recommendations were vague enough that HCWs infected with HIV could litigate to show that they posed no risk and that patients could go to court to show that their providers did.

No patients other than those infected by Acer could claim that they had actually been physically harmed by HIV-positive doctors, of course. Yet many patients, on discovering that their HCWs bore the virus, sued nonetheless. Some of these "AIDS phobia" patients argued that they suffered from the "negligent infliction of emotional distress." (This section relies heavily on the legal research of Scott Burris, a professor and attorney specializing in AIDS law.[75]) In a few cases, courts have allowed patients to sue on the basis that fear of contracting HIV from an HCW is "reasonable." In some instances, the patient was able to collect damages for the period beginning when the patient learned of the "exposure" and ending when it was confirmed that the patient had not contracted the virus.[76] (A negative test six months after the "exposure"' is considered proof that infection did not occur.) In most other cases, the patients typically had to show "proof of actual exposure" to HIV (for example, through a needlestick or cut to the HCW) or at least that they had physical contact with the HCW that created some real possibility of transmitting HIV.[77] Almost no patients will be able to demonstrate such actual exposure; remember, none of Acer's patients knew that they had come into contact with the dentist's blood until they learned that they were infected.

Other patients have argued that the HCWs should have disclosed their HIV status before providing treatment and that because they did not, they violated the patients' right to informed consent. These cases are of two types. In the "negligence" model, a patient can claim that informed consent was not provided only if an injury involving the "concealed" information actually occurs. This has not happened (except for Acer's patients), so these suits have not been successful.[78] In the "battery" model of informed consent, the HCW might be liable for providing care under false pretenses. This would only be the case, however, if the patient specifically asked about the HCW's HIV status as a prerequisite for treatment.[79] Even in this situation, however, the patient's legal prospects are not guaranteed.

The example of Philip Benson illustrates the fragility of both negligence and battery claims. At the height of the HCW and HIV scare—on the day that the CDC announced that at least five dental patients had contracted HIV, and two weeks before Representative Dannemeyer introduced the Kimberly Bergalis Act—Benson, a thirty-nine-year-old obstetrician-gynecologist from Minneapolis, sent letters to 328 of his patients notifying them that he had AIDS and that they should volunteer for HIV tests. According to some of these patients, Benson wore gloves, yet his hands and arms were at times covered with oozing sores.

Among the patients Benson treated was Kathy Nesby. Benson had performed routine gynecological exams on her, delivered her baby, Nicole—after he was diagnosed with AIDS—and continued to provide "well baby" care in which Benson handled the infant. Nesby was horrified at Benson's announcement; when she had asked him about his skin condition, she claimed that he told her it was "an allergic reaction to the sun." Nesby worried that Nicole had "had a diaper rash now for over a month and a half. It's sure taking a long time to clear up." "He takes an oath to save lives, not to give a death sentence," noted another of Benson's patient identified only as "K.A.C."[80]

No death sentences, in fact, were given. None of Benson's patients tested positive for HIV. Still, K.A.C., along with about sixty other patients, sued Benson's estate (in the interim he had died); they claimed "negligent nondisclosure and battery" for the emotional distress they suffered.[81] A lower court dismissed the suit, but the Minnesota Court of Appeals ruled that the patients could take their claims to court. The Minnesota Supreme Court, however, rejected both the negligence and battery claims.[82] As Burris put it, the court ruled in favor of Benson even though Benson "lied to the patient about the reasons for his weight loss and sores on his arm, because he had the patient's consent for the procedure he performed, and his HIV did not significantly increase the risk."[83]

In at least some cases, however, patients treated by HIV-infected HCWs have obtained substantial sums in out-of-court settlements. For example, three other class-action suits have been filed on behalf of more than fifty former patients against another dentist who died of AIDS, with two claims settled for a reported $300,000. In yet another case, a security guard for a hospital obtained a $1.9 million award after he was bitten by a patient with AIDS; the guard had been asked to restrain the patient but had not been notified that the patient was infected. The guard did not become HIV infected as a result of the bite.[84] Still, it appears that courts have not been sympathetic to the claims of patients fearful of contracting HIV from their physicians. And as most attorneys, like Montgomery for Bergalis, take these cases on a contingent-fee basis—that is, they are paid only if they win—the reluctance of courts to make awards surely will make lawyers reluctant to file such cases.

Just as patients have generally been unsuccessful in suing HIV-positive HCWs, infected HCWs have often been thwarted in their attempts at obtaining protection against discrimination. In one common scenario, a hospital—ostensibly trying to avoid the lawsuits of irate patients—will fire or restrict the practice of an HIV-infected HCW. As we have seen, however, persons with HIV fall under the jurisdiction of national disability laws. Accordingly, the HCW's practice can legally be limited only to eliminate a "direct threat" to patient safety.[85] Whether or not an employee creates such a threat depends, as we have seen, on the nature, duration, severity, and probability of the risk. The problem that judges face is that while the likelihood of HIV transmission is extremely low, the perils from infection are extremely high. Some courts have thus sided with the HCWs, noting that the risk of HIV transmission from HCWs is extraordinarily small.[86] Most claims of discrimination by HIV-infected HCWs have been rejected, however, with the courts choosing to emphasize "patients' rights and the supposedly unique and horrible quality of death by AIDS."[87] It appears that the HCWs were especially likely to lose their case if they were doctors, dentists, or nurses providing any care that might be deemed "invasive."

Consider the case of Paul Scoles, a forty-two-year-old orthopedic surgeon when he was diagnosed with HIV in May 1991. One hospital where he practiced, Mercy Catholic Medical Center, concluding that Scoles had been performing exposure-prone procedures, promptly suspended him from operating and obtained a court order to inform his previous patients. A second institution, Graduate Hospital, also made him take a leave of absence.

Scoles sued, claiming that he was discriminated against and that his civil rights had thus been violated.[88] He also filed complaints with the Department of Health and Human Services and the Equal Employment Opportunity Commission. (As a reminder of how powerfully stigmatizing AIDS was, at the time Scoles like many HCWs in such lawsuits was identified only as "John Doe.") He sought reinstatement without restrictions, as well as back pay and punitive damages. In Scoles's eyes,

> I felt that the hospital betrayed me. I worked hard for this hospital for a long time, and they just tossed me out and sent the wolves after me. I just want to get back to practicing, to doing what I'm trained for and what I do fairly well—and that's taking care of people.[89]

As Scoles put it, he sued not only for personal reasons but also to send all hospitals "a clear message that there is a large price to be paid for needlessly destroying the lives and careers of their employees and staff."[90] Indeed, Mercy Catholic's own medical board unanimously recommended that Scoles be reinstated, but the hospital's board of directors rejected this opinion. Scoles's lawyer, Scott Burris, said at the time that the case would be a key test of "how much will the courts rely on medical fact and how much they will rely on irrational fears."[91] The judge ruled in favor of the hospital regarding the core issue of whether it could prohibit Scoles from performing surgery. Still, Mercy Catholic and Scoles reached an out-of-court settlement on other issues deemed "very satisfactory" by Burris.[92]

Ironically, at least one health care worker has successfully sued a patient who exposed her to HIV during an operation but had not told the nurse that she had AIDS.[93] This patient, incidentally, then filed a countersuit against the nurse and her lawyers for invasion of privacy, claiming "malicious disclosure" because they publicized her name rather than referring to her as "Jane Doe."[94]

Have the courts at last satisfactorily settled the legal issues involving patients, health care workers, and HIV? Hardly. Although there have been almost no definitive rulings, the courts seem to be saying two things. To the patients, the message is this: you have no special reason to fear being treated by an HIV-positive health care worker. To the infected HCW, the message is this: your patients have a special reason to fear you, so your employer has the right to restrict your practice. These interpretations are clearly contradictory and, regarding HCWs, misguided. One of the main points of disability discrimination law, after all, is to protect the disabled from discrimination based on fear rather than evidence. That the courts have struggled unsuccessfully with these issues should not be surprising, however, for legal wisdom holds that "hard cases make bad law." The courts, like the CDC, have been unable to resolve neatly the concerns of patients and HCWs. Still, as the CDC, not the courts, bears greatest responsibility for protecting public health, it is to that agency we once again return in the final chapter.

CHAPTER EIGHT

Resolutions
Closing the Acer Case and Preventing Another One

—ᴥᴥᴥ—

his much we know: a Florida dentist and several of his patients have died from AIDS. Each death was a private tragedy, as each person was a son or daughter, a brother or sister, a mother or father. Each person—however infected—had a unique capacity for doing good, for giving love, for feeling suffering. But the accusation that the dentist infected his patients with HIV while providing them medical care also makes this episode a public tragedy. It suggests that patients have reason to be suspicious and fearful of their medical providers. It implies that citizens have cause to doubt their government's ability to guarantee safety in the health care setting. The public distrust of government and the health care system works inevitably to poison public health.

These are deeply troubling prospects because they are, at least in part, true. Health care workers do not provide absolutely safe medical care, nor does the government maintain a risk-free public health system. Yet the poison from this case need not be fatal. Governments and HCWs are already doing much to reduce the risk of HIV transmission in the health care workplace. Together with the patients themselves, they can do more, and do it better, to make medical care safer and more secure. As we consider how these things might improve, let us begin by assessing what the CDC's officials actually did in the case of the Florida dentist.

THE INVESTIGATION: THE CDC WAS RIGHT

Dr. David Acer almost certainly infected Kimberly Bergalis and at least several other patients with HIV while providing them dental care, the CDC concluded. We should be confident that this conclusion is correct. An extensive field investigation by the CDC and Florida's HRS failed to turn up any convincing evidence that Bergalis, Barbara Webb, Lisa Shoemaker, or Sherry Johnson were exposed to HIV outside Acer's clinic. More suspicions can be raised regarding Richard Driskill and John Yecs, who apparently engaged in risky sexual behavior; still, the health officials were unable to confirm that these individuals had come into intimate contact with other HIV-positive persons. And while the field investigation helped to eliminate other sources of infection, the CDC's genetic research showed that all six patients shared a common viral "signature" with Acer. Taken together, the field and genetic studies established overwhelming evidence that Acer infected his patients.

The CDC also concluded that it did not know exactly how Acer infected these patients. We, too, should be ambivalent. There is the strongest evidence that Acer did not transmit HIV to these patients through sexual contact. It is also virtually impossible that he infected the patients by using accidentally contaminated equipment. It is more likely, although it still seems virtually unimaginable, that Acer spread the virus by accidentally injuring himself and bleeding directly into the patients' mouths. HIV can be spread this way, yet any dentist infecting six patients this way would have to be both incompetent and unlucky. Acer might have murdered his patients, yet the only evidence for this is the improbability of the other potential causes. Although each of us might have a hunch about how the infections occurred, ultimately that is all we have.

The CDC surely considered whether Acer had a motive to kill his patients and whether his patients had incentives to lie about their infections. Let us now consider the motives that the CDC and other participants had in this affair. As with Acer himself, we can only speculate about what really motivated the public officials—Curran, Jaffe,

Ciesielski, Economou, and the rest. These officials, for their part, would deny that they had any motive other than finding the truth. It is hard to see how they obtained any private gain by identifying Acer as the source of the infection. It is easy to imagine, moreover, that their lives would have been much easier if they had determined that the patients had *not* been infected by Acer. By concluding that Acer infected Bergalis and the others, these officials incurred the wrath of the public for "letting" it happen and from medical professionals for fostering public hysteria. To these officials, however, the controversy and the headaches are part of their work. Their regrets are that individuals became infected with HIV and died, not that their jobs have become more difficult as a result. Even after reading the "Dear Nikki" letter publicized nationwide, Economou remarked, "It doesn't matter what our people went through. It pales in comparison to what Kimberly goes through."[1]

Consider, next, the CDC's admission that it does not know how the infections occurred. If the CDC officials wanted to live a simpler life, they might have concluded that Acer had murdered his patients. The professionals might have been relieved, as this conclusion would suggest that no new medical policies were needed. Patients might have been soothed, as this then would have been just one more mass murder, to which our society seems hardened. An innocent man would perhaps have been falsely condemned, but it is alas doubtful that many protests would have been raised on Acer's behalf.

In contrast, if the CDC officials had wanted merely to increase their authority, they might have preferred to identify contaminated equipment as the cause of the infection. If dirty tools were to blame, then the CDC, the professionals, and the public could all have avoided difficult dilemmas. Acer's practice could just have been portrayed as "lax" in its infection control—which it apparently was. A nice technical solution would exist for preventing future infections from infected equipment: sterilize it. There would be some additional cost and effort for doing this, of course, but it would not have pitted health care workers against patients (and both against the CDC). The CDC, moreover, could have relied on well-respected methods of infection control to solve the problem.

If the CDC wanted to maintain its prestige, it at least needed to arrive at *some* definitive conclusion about the cause of the infections. The most difficult judgment for the CDC to make was the one that it actually made: that the cause of the infection was unknown. This conclusion must have been personally difficult for the CDC's officials for a couple of reasons. In an age where every empirical problem is assumed to have an answer, it raises questions about their competence: "How could they not find out how it happened? Don't they know what they're doing?" Lacking information about how the infections occurred also made it infinitely more difficult to develop policy: how can they prevent the recurrence of an event when they do not even know what caused it?

If the conclusions that Acer infected the patients in an unknown manner made the CDC officials' lives more difficult and if they reaped no personal or professional benefits from these conclusions, then why did they make them? For the cynical among us who assume that public officials always act in their own self-interest, this should be a difficult question. The answer is more easily apparent to those with a less jaundiced view of public life: perhaps the officials actually did want to determine the truth as best they could. As a matter of professional ethics, these public health officials believed they were responsible for learning how the infections occurred. Moreover, these officials preferred to report these results honestly, making conclusions where the evidence supported them and expressing ambivalence where the data were unclear. Finally, the officials reported the results because they believed the results were important for *public health* (and not their own careers). In this view, the public needed to know the conclusions in all their ambiguity. It is worth considering, then, that the CDC made an honest attempt to promote the public health as best it could—in other words, that it was largely motivated by the "public spirit."[2]

It is hard to see how it was in the personal interest of the CDC officials to make the conclusions that they did. But what about the motivations of the others involved? CIGNA and CNA, the companies sued by the patients, had strong and clear financial incentives to prove that Acer was not the source of the infection. The CIGNA and CNA representatives were not hired to identify the truth or to protect the public health; they were hired as advocates to save CIGNA and CNA money in the lawsuits. It is noteworthy that even with this monetary incentive, the companies' representatives were unable to find evidence that convincingly contradicted the CDC's conclusions regarding Acer's culpability.

Members of the media, too, had personal and professional reasons to prove the CDC wrong. If they did—or at least if they presented a plausible case—they would win notoriety, airtime, and maybe even a Pulitzer Prize. This does not mean that reporters have a motive to lie. Like the CDC's officials, reporters, too, have professional incentives to get the story right. Yet if they do, and the story agrees with the CDC, then in the eyes of the media there is no story. No reporter gets ahead by merely confirming that official sources are accurate. Not surprisingly, some of the biggest stories about the Bergalis case (such as the ones implying that she had contracted HIV through sex or that Acer had deliberately infected his patients) were based on skimpier information and greater speculation than the official reports. Yet journalists and private detectives found out nothing material about the patients' infections that the public officials had not already discovered. Private money did not generate better information than did professional duty.

Other governmental organizations had their own motivations to show that the CDC's conclusions were incorrect. Late in 1990, Democratic congressman Ted Weiss, skeptical of the CDC's conclusions in the Florida dentist case, requested that the GAO conduct an inquiry into the CDC's handling of it. This was not the first time that Weiss had asked the GAO to investigate the CDC and its involvement in AIDS research. The GAO and the CDC indeed had a history of contentious relations over AIDS policy and programs dating back to the early years of the epidemic, and this animosity spilled over into the inquiry of the Florida dentist.[3] Part of the enmity between the two agencies was institutional, as the GAO works for Congress within the legislative branch while the CDC serves the president in the executive branch. Partisan differences contributed to the tension; at the time of this case, Republicans controlled the White House and Democrats ruled the Congress. Although the GAO and the CDC were both federal agencies, the CDC had no reason to expect the GAO would go easy on it.

As the principal investigator of that GAO investigation, I began the study expecting to find that the CDC had made major mistakes in its work. The GAO culture supported this expectation. As the congressional "watchdog," the GAO encourages its employees to seek evidence of governmental failure and has built its reputation upon finding it. As George Silberman, my boss, put it neatly: "If we come up with a finding that the CDC is wrong, our careers are made. There are lots of incentives in the [GAO] and outside of the organization for us to come up with a finding that its skeptical of the [CDC's] conclusions."[4] Yet despite these incentives, the GAO report concluded that the CDC's "investigation as a whole was found to have been both thorough and competent."[5] The only reason that the GAO reached this conclusion was that it believed the CDC was right.

The CDC public officials were thus willing to admit that they did not know what happened even though other observers claimed that they did. The CDC officials acknowledge forthrightly that they do not know how Bergalis and the other patients were infected. This must not have been an easy admission, but it is clearly an honest one. While it is easy to speculate publicly—as many have—about how Acer *might* have infected his patients, in fact no one truly knows. Life is not a Sherlock Holmes story. Some mysteries are truly unsolvable.

If the CDC's conclusions are hard to fault, its efforts to reach them seem easier to criticize. The most serious criticisms are that the CDC treated Acer too generously and Bergalis too harshly. Based on the motivations, training, experiences, and beliefs of the CDC investigators, both claims are probably true. CDC officials were skeptical, as they should have been, toward Bergalis's claims; they were credulous, as they need not have been, of Acer's position.

One irony is that while the CDC has pledged to question HCWs more closely in the future regarding HIV transmission, it has offered no suggestions about its future treatment of investigated patients. Perhaps it should. As we saw in Chapter Two, the Bergalis family came to see the CDC as an enemy rather than an advocate. This situation cannot be entirely reversed, but the CDC—along with every other agency—might benefit by considering in each circumstance how its interests align with those of the citizens with which it deals. The CDC was obligated to examine Kimberly Bergalis's claims thoroughly, but had it done so as a sympathetic partner rather than as a hostile inquisitor, it could have come to the same conclusion with less bitterness.

WHO SHOULD MAKE POLICY?

The hardest question remains: Could the CDC have done a better job of crafting policies to lower the risk and reduce the fear of HIV transmission in medical settings? We can think about answering this question in a couple of ways. We could first try to develop an ideal set of policy proposals and then consider how the CDC could have been persuaded to adopt them. Alternately, we could try to design an ideal way to develop policies and then consider how this process could lead to appropriate policies. In other words, we can begin either with policy substance or with political process.

Almost everyone involved in this case has emphasized policies and decried politics. Experts and patients alike have insisted that the policies they favor are the best ones and that if not for "politics," these policies would be adopted. But as should by now be clear, because policies for HIV and HCWs involve public health ("How do we make the health care workplace safer?"), economics ("What are the most efficient ways to make the workplace safer? How much should we spend to do so?"), ethics ("Whose rights should be protected? What are the responsibilities of HCWs and patients?"), and law ("Which policies are constitutional? Which are legal?"), there is simply no correct answer to the basic question of what our policies should be. All answers have various costs and benefits and will harm certain people while helping others.

Indeed, focusing solely on the policy questions has hindered attempts to develop solutions, as there is no analytical way to resolve the questions. How much risk is too much? How much should we spend to save a life? Whose rights should take precedence—the patients' right to know or the HCWs' right to privacy? Because there is no objective way to answer these questions, the methods used to address them become critically important. These methods do not provide easy solutions either, as was evident from the fact that experts and patients at times vehemently disagreed about which policies are best. The Bergalis family and the HIV-positive HCWs, along with the other partisans for each side, may never lie down together like the lion and the lamb—nor be able to agree on which of them is in which role, for that matter. Yet through politics, it might still be possible to develop policies that obtain more general support from the broader public, the professional communities, and even from the most fervent advocates themselves.

Before we consider how the policy decisions should be reached, it is perhaps helpful to reconsider who actually has made policy regarding HIV and health care workers. By now it should be clear that this issue has two responses: everyone and no one. Legislatures, courts, and public health agencies at the national, state, and local level have all "made policy" by enacting laws, making rulings, or issuing regulations or guidelines. These policies, considered together, have not finally resolved the matter, creating instead a mixture of rulings that are ambiguous or contradictory. There is still no policy consensus, for example, concerning which health care workers, in which situations, must determine their HIV status or disclose it to which patients.

It might be tempting, then, to conclude that *someone* should have the power and responsibility for making authoritative policy decisions for HIV. There is indeed a long tradition in the United States of thinking that policy conflicts should be ended through administrative means, of believing that policy problems would be solved if only our government had the proper structure. Sandra Panem's book *The AIDS Bureaucracy*, one of the few serious attempts to prescribe how AIDS policy should be made and not just what it should be, embodies this wish. As Panem would have it, epidemics such as AIDS would be greatly eased if "responsibility and leadership" were "centralized and assigned to a federal official" having "generous and centralized finances" and a "flexible budget." This official would then use "central oversight and management" and "immediate, short-term, and long-term . . . strategic planning" to address—and presumably control—the epidemic.[6]

These recommendations, as attractive as they might sound, deserve close scrutiny. Who, after all, favors splintered authority, rigid and inadequate budgets, and myopic plans? No one—although it is true that other observers argue that the best way to address public problems is to decentralize authority and impose tight controls over governmental spending; these are respectable ideas, but exactly the opposite of what Panem recommends. Moreover, a call for "long-term strategic planning" begs the central question of what the strategy should be.

Even if centralized authority seemed useful in theory, it cannot be consistently applied in fact. As policy problems overlap, it is not actually possible to have centralized and specialized authority over each problem. As Panem points out, addressing the AIDS epidemic requires medical research and public education, for example. But tuberculosis is another major public health problem, and dealing with it also requires medical research and education. If authority over AIDS is centralized in one office and tuberculosis is centralized in another, then the research or education efforts for each disease would be separated from the other. This would mean duplication of effort and failure to coordinate resources, for instance—the very things that Panem seeks to avoid. One could, of course, centralize medical research over both diseases in one office and place health education in another—but then *these* functions would be separated from each other. Unless all policy authority is centralized in a single office ("The Bureau of Everything"), the problem of divided but overlapping jurisdictions cannot be resolved.

But Americans have an historical preference for decentralized government, so let us take it as a given that national, state, and local legislatures, agencies, and courts are all likely to be involved in making policy for HIV and HCWs, as we have seen. Even in this highly fragmented situation, however, it is possible to draw lessons for the future by reviewing how policy was made in the past.

This was the pattern: Congress began to make policy on the HIV issue partly because the CDC had not. OSHA based its policies, to a great extent, on the CDC guidelines. The courts have been influenced by the recommendations of the CDC. The states had to develop their own policies based on those offered by the CDC. In short, even though numerous governmental institutions have made policies for HIV in the health care workplace, many, if not most of them, have turned to the CDC for guidance. Even though the CDC was no centralized authority, the other governmental institutions looked to that agency for its health policy guidance. The CDC remains the best choice as the appropriate "who" for making health policy for HIV and HCWs.

How Should Decisions Be Reached?

That the CDC was the most sensible agency for making policy does not necessarily imply that sensible policy was made. By all accounts, the CDC mishandled the job. But just what does this mean? Does it mean that because the CDC did not call for mandatory testing and patient notification, more patients have been infected from HIV-positive health care workers? As far as we can tell, the answer is no; there have been no other documented cases of HIV transmission from health care worker to patient in this country since Acer closed his clinic. Does it mean that because the CDC did call for HIV-positive HCWs who conduct exposure-prone procedures to seek advice from expert panels, infected HCWs have been driven from practice? The answer here, regrettably, is a less definite no. By the summer of 1996, almost fifty HIV-positive HCWs had called the Gay and Lesbian Medical Association (GLMA) to report that they had been fired after their HIV status became known, with almost another one hundred reporting various other incidents of workplace discrimination. (The GLMA considers these reports "the tip of the iceberg."[7]) Still, to the best of our knowledge, no additional patients have been infected, and the vast majority of HIV-infected health care workers have continued to use their medical expertise to assist patients. By these criteria, the CDC guidelines should be judged at least a qualified success. That no one has been satisfied with the policies, even though their consequences seem mainly to have met their goals, suggests that the discontent arises more from the process than from the results.

Ironically, advocates of both the patient and the expert viewpoints agree on two things. First, the policies would have been better if the CDC had shown real "leadership." Second, the CDC needed to be removed from "politics" in order to protect the public health better. The clear implication is that if the CDC had real leaders, it would have done the right thing—namely, whatever each side wanted done. Furthermore, without political interference, the CDC would have been free to do either the "moral" thing—that is, to identify and remove HIV-positive HCWs from medical practice—or the "scientific" thing—that is, not to take action against these people unless they posed a demonstrated risk of infecting patients. The advocates thus defined leadership as "decisive support for my position" and apolitical as "action in agreement with my view." Experts and patients alike appear to believe that the leaders of an apolitical CDC would adopt their favored policies.

These beliefs reveal a fundamental misunderstanding of health policy and a limited view of leadership. Health policy is inherently political—AIDS policy is not unique in this respect—so it is impossible to make the CDC apolitical. To be sure, AIDS is often called the most "political" disease in history, but this is incorrect. All diseases are political in that citizens and governments decide what kinds of actions will be taken by whom and at whose expense and profit. AIDS is, however, perhaps the most "democratic" disease, in that those affected by it have voiced their opinions and expected governments to respond to them.

The CDC in this case needed to decide who could perform what kinds of medical procedures under which conditions; it needed to decide what kinds of risks and burdens would be faced by health care workers and by patients. How could this be done in an apolitical way? Through science? No: science provides evidence but cannot make decisions. Moreover, science itself is political in that it requires choices about methods, evidence, and interpretations. Research might tell us the probabilities of HIV transmission by health care workers (although, as we have seen, different methods provide different estimates), but it cannot tell us whether these risks are too high to accept. Through philosophy? No: logic might help clarify our thinking regarding the ideal relationship between physicians and patients, for instance, but it cannot tell us whose rights are more important or precisely how to balance competing rights. There is no computer that we can program, no algorithm we can compose, no sage we can consult, that will help us to make health policy in an apolitical fashion.

It is no small irony that while vilifying politics, the advocates of patient and expert views have themselves been highly political. Kimberly Bergalis herself was no stranger to political action. She and her family learned how to use the mass media to promote her cause. Her "Dear Nikki" letter ("If laws are not formed to provide [patients] protection, then my suffering and death were in vain") was not sent to HRS investigator Economou but to the press.[8] Bergalis appeared on numerous talk shows calling for mandatory testing and patient notification. She testified before a congressional committee in support of the "Kimberly Bergalis Act." Those who oppose her position have been no less aggressive in trying to influence the policy debates. Each advocate took political action because it wanted its position to prevail.

Those who want the CDC to be apolitical also misunderstand history. Health policy never has been, nor can it be, without politics. Even a cursory examination of the history of health policy shows that public health has always been a controversial topic. Every epidemic is marked by the sharpest differences of opinion concerning causes and treatments. AIDS may be different from any other contagious disease, but every contagion is the same in that each produces strong sentiments about what the government should do.

If it is impossible to remove policy from politics, then what kind of leadership did the CDC need? Both patients and experts wanted a leader who would implement their preferences. This implies that a leader must ignore opposing views. Is this what each side really wants? Perhaps—if it could be guaranteed that the leader would favor *your* views. But what if this cannot be assured? What if a leader is to be selected for the CDC and neither side knew for certain this person's preferences? Unless each side wants to roll the dice in a game of winner-take-all, it is reasonable that both sides will want a leader who will take their views seriously as policy is developed. Each side might also want ways to ensure that its views, in particular, are taken seriously.

Each side might thus seek to ensure that the leader's powers are limited. Each side, in other words, might want to have the kind of leaders that the CDC actually had.[9]

Paradoxically, uncompromising leadership would have weakened the CDC. After all, the CDC has the power only to advise, not command. If its leader had decreed that a mandatory testing and patient notification program be adopted, it would probably have inspired widespread noncompliance—and resistance—among health professionals. If its leader had simply proclaimed that patients need not worry about HIV in the medical setting, the public would likely have lost confidence in the CDC as its advocate. As Burris sensibly sees it, "health measures that inspire serious resistance among their objects are health measures that will not work."[10]

But there is another kind of leader: one who attempts to unite disparate factions, to find points of consensus, and to develop compromises. Curran, for example, argues that leaders at the CDC *must* engage both the public and the experts in the policy process if their leadership is to be effective. The participants in the HIV debate might accordingly ask themselves, Would we want the CDC leadership to ignore our claims for action?

It does seem clear that the participants were willing to have the views of the *other* side ignored. Patients' advocates appeared eager to dismiss the expertise of the medical community as merely selfish. Experts, in turn, seemed willing at times to reject the beliefs of the public as irrational. Given the passion with which these political views were held, we might well consider that the CDC's attempts to bring the parties together to find a common solution demonstrated the very essence of leadership.

The challenge, then, was for the CDC to develop its guidelines in such a way that advocates on all sides believed that their interests had been taken seriously and that they were being treated fairly. In other words, the CDC's leadership faced the challenge of resolving conflict. Yet without the help of their constituents, leaders can only suppress conflict. To reconcile conflicts, leaders must help the participants themselves find ways to settle their problems.

Several steps appear to be especially useful in doing this.[11] A first step is to recognize explicitly that conflict exists. Surely the participants in this case must already be aware of this. But not necessarily. In the transcripts of the CDC's two open meetings to discuss the need for new guidelines, no one—and in particular no CDC official—

plainly says, "There are major disagreements about what the guidelines should be. The public wants us to test health care workers and reveal the results to patients. Health care workers believe that such actions would harm health care workers without improving public health." Such a simple statement at least makes clear the core differences that exist; it also reminds the disputants that they and the CDC face tough challenges in settling these disagreements.

Even though the CDC did not make the conflict explicit, it at least did one valuable—although no doubt painful—thing to bring the conflict to the surface. The CDC brought a wide variety of interests and organizations with differing appetites to the table. By doing this the CDC let the conflict bubble up. While it is unlikely that medical professionals enjoyed this ("What are all these lawyers, union representatives, and activists doing at a public *health* meeting?"), these newcomers could appropriately reply that it was a *public* health meeting. The CDC can no longer, if it ever could, hope to issue recommendations on controversial topics without bringing a broad spectrum of the public into the process. Recognizing conflict requires this.

A second step is to obtain agreement from the participants that they want to resolve the conflict. This might sound obvious: doesn't everyone want a resolution? Not really, at least if the resolution does not give them exactly what they want. The American political system actually encourages such thinking because it provides so many places to influence policy and appeal decisions. Why work with the CDC to resolve the issues if you think you can get a better deal from the Congress? Why accept the congressional or regulatory decision if you can take it to court? Why accept the court's interpretation of the law if you can get the law changed?

The American Dental Association, for example, had ample time and opportunity to make its views known to OSHA over the five years it was developing its regulations. The ADA nonetheless did not accept OSHA's decisions as binding and so sued for relief. This might be called "wanting to resolve the conflict but only if the conflict is resolved to your complete satisfaction." Consider also the medical associations' response to the CDC guidelines. The American Medical Association and the American Dental Association, in particular, led the CDC to believe that they agreed to the idea of developing lists of exposure-prone medical procedures. (These lists were essential for the guidelines to have any real meaning.) Yet after the guidelines were issued, both organizations backtracked on their pledges. As much as anything, the inability of the medical organizations to follow through was responsible for the collapse of the guidelines. To be fair, there are good reasons for opposing such lists, and these organizations no doubt also struggled to decide what kinds of measures were appropriate. My point is that the medical groups should have pressed these reasons as forcibly as possible while the guidelines were being developed, not afterward. The CDC, lacking enforcement powers, cannot compel participants to agree to its guidelines or even pledge to agree. It can hardly even publicize the fact that these organizations retreated on their commitments. Yet it seems perverse, at least for these organizations, to criticize the CDC as lacking the leadership necessary to develop satisfactory recommendations.

Perhaps the most important step in resolving conflict, one that might have been assisted by CDC officials but cannot be taken by them, is to get the participants to develop a real understanding of the issues from the others' perspective. In most conflicts, and this one was no exception, this step is not taken by those demanding policy change. As Marcus describes it:

> Conflict is . . . a process of simplification. We ignore the reasons, justifications, viewpoints, and concerns of the other side. We dismiss the texture of their statements, and we are blind to the weaknesses of our own. They are wrong and we are right. Their problem is without merit; ours is valid.[12]

Truly understanding the views of one's apparent opponents is never easy, and when the issues involve life and livelihood, as they did here, the job is even more difficult. But health care workers, for their part, should be able to understand the patients' point of view. After all, almost all HCWs are also patients from time to time. As professionals, HCWs know that the risks of HIV transmission in the health care setting are extremely low. As persons, however, HCWs themselves often fear being infected.[13] Anyone who doubts this simply has to ask any health care worker, "Would it worry you to let your spouse or your child undergo an invasive procedure by an HIV-infected health care worker?" Surely professionals should also be able to empathize with their patients' fears.

It is harder for the public to see through the eyes of the experts or, especially, through those of HIV-infected HCWs. It is difficult enough to imagine what it is like to learn you are infected. (It is a terrible fact that the suicide rate jumps among those persons diagnosed HIV positive.[14]) When Bergalis's doctor brought in her test results, but before he had told her, Kimberly recalled, "I, I knew, and then I started having, you know, chills in my feet and all the way up my body and I just started . . . and I started trembling and crying. Am I going to die?"[15] She wrote down her thoughts:

> I just found out a few minutes ago that I do have AIDS. I'm so scared. I have to now tell my parents & sisters. I . . . just want to close my eyes & open them & see that this is all a mistake—a horrible nightmare. I want to leave this hospital—I want to just run and go back to being a little girl again. . . . I'm trembling & I can't help it. I'm so scared. . . . I just don't know how much more I can take. Please pray for me.[16]

And, as we have seen, Bergalis surely understood how painful it was to tell others—even HCWs—about the diagnosis, as she herself hid it from her own dentist. Acer's other patients no doubt sympathized with Kimberly. After Sherry Johnson held a press conference to announce that she was the sixth infected patient, her stepmother, reflecting on the hostility shown other persons with AIDS, stated that "we didn't know if our home would be standing when we got back."[17] Can we not all also sympathize with these fears and desires? But are they not the same as those felt by infected HCWs, who just want to run back to the time before they were infected, to be able to live their lives as they had planned, not to have patients scream or kick them out of their jobs? Can we not all at least imagine that if we were infected, we would want others to allow us to continue to live our lives—and to do our jobs—as much as possible as we did before?

The question posed to the health care workers might thus be usefully reversed. Patients might ask themselves, "If my spouse or my child or I were infected and needed an invasive procedure, would I expect HCWs to provide care?" The humane and human answer must be "yes." A person might equivocate by saying that "I expect *some* HCW to provide me care, but HCWs ultimately should have the choice whether or not to do so." In many cases—such as when emergency care is needed, and only one emergency room is available—this answer would not be relevant. Many people might rightly declare that this question is altogether hypothetical because they are at essentially no risk for being infected (as they do not engage in any risky behaviors). These people, as a result, cannot imagine posing a risk to the health care workers because they were infected. But this response mirrors the one given by infected HCWs who claim that they pose no measurable risk of infecting their patients. What patients and HCWs each seem to be saying is that my risk of infecting you is too small to worry about.

WHAT SHOULD THE POLICIES BE?

A next task is for the participants—patients, experts, CDC—to find their common interests in resolving the conflict. It is possible that these interests can exist even among blood enemies (who, for their own entirely selfish reasons, might still prefer a cease-fire over continued hostilities). But the possibility for a common interest to emerge is much higher if the participants are truly able to envision the aspirations and fears of the others so that all may ask such basic questions as "How might we best obey the Golden Rule?" or "'How might we do for others as we would have them do for us?"

The argument that mandatory HIV testing and disclosure cannot achieve the Golden Rule is strong and has been considered in detail elsewhere. Still, a brief summary, focusing on the moral dimensions, may highlight the main issues. First, we need to recognize that all lives have equal moral worth and so are equally worth protecting. This suggests that we should be concerned about protecting equally all persons, patients as well as HCWs, from all threats in the health care setting. This idea implies that if HCWs are to be tested, then so should those who seek treatment; if the professionals must disclose their HIV status, then so should their patients. Let us add the premise that both patients and providers are equal in their desire to protect their own lives.

These premises have two main implications for testing and disclosure. First, almost everyone will perceive that everybody else should be tested and should disclose the test results. Patients and HCWs alike will generally want to know whether the other person is infected with HIV. But it is not possible to gain this knowledge, and it is costly to try. It is literally impossible to know if someone is infected with HIV, given the current technology, until some time after a person has become infected. So the patient or HCW cannot be certain that the other person is uninfected, even if each person is tested immediately before the treatment is performed. This is of more than theoretical concern. Every time an invasive procedure takes place, blood is potentially exposed. Unless both parties have tested negative for HIV repeatedly, and neither party has had even a potential exposure to HIV since the last test, then neither party can be secure in the knowledge that the other person is not infected.

So it is often the case that the patient or the health care worker cannot know whether the other has been tested and found to be uninfected. The health care worker, for example, must often provide emergency treatment, in which case there is no time to test. The patient, on the other hand, typically receives treatment from a health care professional who is frequently exposed to blood, so there is no way to ensure that this professional has not been exposed to HIV-contaminated blood. Requiring both patients and HCWs to be tested for HIV could certainly identify most persons who are infected. But it is a fantasy to think that all patients or health care workers could be identified by testing.

It is to no one's advantage to treat, or to receive treatment from, other persons who are infected with HIV. Health care workers clearly understand that if they are identified as being infected with HIV, their patients will leave them and they will lose their livelihood (as they move toward losing their life). On the other hand, HCWs have their own selfish reasons to abandon any patient who acknowledges being infected. Yet if patients or health care workers avoid contact with HIV-infected persons, the only conclusion that can be drawn is that infected persons will neither be able to obtain nor provide much health care. This outcome would be morally acceptable only if we accept that persons will be prevented from obtaining health care precisely when they need it most.

How might we best improve the safety of *both* patients and providers in the health care setting? Let us consider, for a moment, the possibilities. What if either patient or provider were infected, but neither knew which one it was? In this case, both persons would surely insist that the best possible infection control procedures—in other words, universal precautions—be used. This choice "from behind the veil of ignorance," in which neither person knows with certainty the relevant information, accurately describes most interactions between patients and HCWs because it is impossible for either person to know with certainty that the other is *not* infected with the virus.[18] Furthermore, if both patient and provider were known to be infected with HIV, or if neither actually were infected, then universal precautions would still provide the best means to prevent transmission of HIV and every other infection between HCW and patient. In short, universal precautions provide the best protection against *all* infections in the health care setting for the *vast majority* of patient-provider contacts. For these reasons, the CDC's promotion of universal guidelines seems especially helpful for public health.

The toughest cases, of course, are those in which either the patient or the provider knows that the other one is infected. If the provider knows the patient is infected, can this knowledge be used to improve the provider's safety *and* the patient's care? Most experts say no. If universal precautions are already being used, it is not clear how this information could be beneficially used by both parties. The HCW, to be sure, could use this information for private gain by refusing to provide care. Can patients profitably use the knowledge that a provider is HIV positive to improve the quality of their health care? Not if they plan to stick with that provider. If they do, patients should expect their HCWs to use universal precautions to protect everyone. The only way this information could "improve" the patient's care is if the patient deserts the HIV-positive provider. I've put "improve" in quotation marks because the patient cannot know in advance that switching from a health care provider known to be HIV positive to another one will actually improve the treatment. Switching will remove one infinitesimally small risk but will introduce others of unknown magnitude.

What are the common interests regarding patient notification? At the outset, there might once again seem to be no mutual interests, as patients might generally want to know whether their HCW is infected and the HCWs might generally be reluctant to reveal such information. But it might be possible to devise policies that respect both these views. Again, these policies would oppose adopting either the public's preference for mandatory disclosure or the professionals' rejection of required notification. These recommendations would also rely to a greater extent on ethical standards than legal ones. The disadvantages of establishing purely legal standards are that they typically build "floors" ("I broke no law") rather than create "ceilings" ("I did the right thing") and that they promote adversarial relationships rather than cooperative ones.

Here is how such a policy might look. Regarding patients, the CDC could have stated,

> We strongly believe that patients should learn as much as possible about their physical condition and medical care so that they may take

steps to lead healthier lives. We therefore encourage patients to ask their physicians *any* questions they believe relevant to their condition or care. Patients must ultimately have the final say regarding the care they receive.

This statement serves two main purposes relevant not only to HIV but to all other medical problems. First, it informs patients that there is a clear link between knowledge and health and that people who know more about their health and health care tend to be healthier. Second, it reestablishes the principle that the patient is sovereign in the health care setting and allows the patient to decide which matters are relevant to his or her decisions about care.

The idea that patients are sovereign in the health care setting is morally attractive and legally sound. The U.S. Supreme Court has affirmed the right of patients to refuse treatment, even if the physician believes this decision is unsound or irrational:

"No right is held more sacred, or is more carefully guarded, by the common law, than the right of every individual to the possession and control of his own person, free from all restraint or interference of others." . . . The principle that a competent person has a constitutionally protected liberty interest in refusing unwanted medical treatment may be inferred from our prior decisions.[19]

The insistence that HCWs do not have a duty to disclose when they are HIV positive because they do not have to disclose the other greater risks they might pose to patients (through their alcohol or substance abuse, for example, or because they have had a series of malpractice judgments against them) seems especially weak. HCWs cannot describe (or even know) all the risks that they might pose for patients. But rather than concluding that this relieves HCWs of their obligations to inform their patients, it suggests that patients can and should ask about these other risk factors. Physicians are trained to ask questions to learn about their patients' illnesses. It is now time to encourage patients to ask questions to learn more about their HCWs' competencies.

Patients should insist that the medical providers answer these questions in terms that they understand. In particular, patients might ask about the HCWs' infection control procedures. If universal precautions are the main defense against infection, patients have special reason to expect their HCWs to use them rigorously and vigorously. Ask, for example, "How do you sterilize your equipment?" Virtually everything should be heat-treated or disposable. "How do I know you do sterilize properly?" Your HCW should typically put on a new pair of disposable gloves in your presence and open sealed sterile packages containing any tools to be used.

The CDC might also have provided some advice to HCWs about how to answer the disclosure question. It might have reminded them, for example, that a health care professional has the duty to provide patients with the best possible medical care. This care includes the information that will help the patient make a well-informed choice regarding treatment. The CDC might have suggested that if a patient asks you directly whether you are HIV-positive, you might respond that "extensive medical studies have shown that the risk of patients becoming infected with HIV through medical care, whether or not their providers are infected, is remote. I use the infection control techniques that reduce the risk of all infections to the lowest level practical." This statement would serve a couple of purposes. In the first place, it provides the information regarding objective risk that a strong majority of the medical community has deemed most relevant for patients to know. Yet it also provides the personal commitment—a promise—from the HCWs to provide the safest possible care to the sovereign patients. Parenthetically, the use of the word *remote* is intended to convey that in legal terms, the risk is not "significant."

Many patients would probably be educated and relieved by the providers' suggested answers; after all, the patients' real concern should be that their HCW will not harm them, not whether their HCW has some personal characteristic. Some patients, no doubt, would not be satisfied with that answer and so would persist in seeking a yes or no response. The provider, having given the appropriate medical information, need not feel an obligation to reveal this personal information. If the patient is not satisfied with this answer, then he or she has the power to choose another provider. Admittedly, as more and more patients enter into managed care insurance systems that limit their ability to choose their providers, the ability of patients to shop around for satisfactory answers may be limited to what the patients are willing to pay. But this is a reminder that all medical choices have consequences and that no choices are completely free.

Like any set of recommendations, most HCWs would need to adopt them in order for them to be effective. If only the HIV-positive

HCWs give the recommended answer, while HCWs who believe themselves to be uninfected answer, "No, I am not HIV positive," then giving the recommended answer would be tantamount to acknowledging infection. Patients would then flee the practices of these HCWs.

But HCWs have a common interest in providing this recommended answer for themselves as well as their patients. In the first place, no HCWs who are routinely exposed to patients' blood can truthfully claim to *know* that they are not infected with HIV. Moreover, all HCWs who perform invasive procedures must understand that they could be infected with HIV someday and so should consider carefully not only what answer seems to be in their self-interest now but which one might be in their interest in the future. Finally, no HCW can truthfully answer the question that underlies the patients' real concern: "Can you guarantee me that this medical procedure will heal me, not harm me?" No health care worker can make this guarantee. HCWs can, at best, provide historical and statistical information about risks and pledge to do their best to heal the patient.

Patients and the medical community also have a common interest in the competency of the providers. Patients thus have the right to expect that their HCWs will be competent. HCWs, for their part, have a moral, legal, and professional duty to practice only if they are competent. Obsessive focus on a provider's HIV status can only serve to distract attention from the broader and more important issue of competency of care.

One could assert that HIV-positive dentists or surgeons are inherently incompetent to provide care. This is an odd definition of competence. Competence might be better assessed by observing performance. Consider two tests. First, imagine that skilled judges observed a large group of HCWs, some of whom were HIV positive, as they provided patient care. Is it possible for the judges to identify the infected providers merely by watching them provide care? No, it is not, although the judges could rate the competence of the providers by observing the skill with which they dispensed care. Second, imagine that the judges did not watch the providers perform but instead inspected the patients' outcomes. Is it possible that the judges could identify the HIV-positive HCWs on the basis of the patients' health after the procedures? It is possible but extremely unlikely that at least one of the infected HCWs could be identified in this test. Still, there is little reason to think that the patients of the infected HCWs will have worse outcomes than those the other HCWs. It is certain, in fact, that there would be many more bad outcomes—death, disfigure-ment, pain—among those HCWs who were *not* HIV positive. (If 1 percent of HCWs are HIV positive, then there are ninety-nine unin-fected HCWs for each infected one. This means that unless HIV-pos-itive HCWs are ninety-nine times more dangerous than uninfected HCWs—and there is no evidence to suggest that they are—more patients will be hurt by uninfected HCWs than infected ones.) Given that neither competence test could be used by our skilled judges to identify the HIV-positive HCWs, we cannot conclude that infected HCWs are any less competent as a result of their infection than their peers. Concluding that any group of HCWs is incompetent, even though no skill-based tests shows this to be the case, is mere prejudice.

Focusing on *competence,* rather than HIV status, can provide ben-efits for both the public and the medical community. The profession-als, for their part, can demonstrate their seriousness at improving public health by calling more vigorously for competence reviews of their peers and sanctions against those who prove inept. The AMA and the ADA, with their call for a "no identifiable risk" standard, appear particularly weak on this point. Far better for the AMA and the ADA to state that it will strive to produce the highest possible level of competence among *all* its members—not just the HIV-positive ones—through training, surveillance, and disciplinary actions. Not only would this improve the quality of health care but it would also provide a clear signal to the public that the professionals are neither indifferent to its concerns nor willing to offer it scapegoats (in the form of HIV-positive HCWs). Public confidence in health care providers, an important component of successful medical care, would be enhanced by a vigorous focus on competence. Monitoring and improving competence are no simple tasks, certainly, but they are ones that must constantly be emphasized.[20]

HIV-positive HCWs, to be sure, will also be affected by a renewed emphasis on competence. Infected HCWs face the prospect—as do all HCWs—that their skills will decline as time passes. Knowing firsthand the horrors of infection, they should be especially sensitive to the pos-sibility that they could infect others. It is incumbent on infected HCWs—as with all HCWs—that they restrict their practices as their competence declines. It might be easy for many individuals to ignore signs of this decline. As a result, those HCWs who are HIV positive have a special reason, for their own health as well as the health of their patients, to seek appropriate medical care (including an assessment of physical and mental competence for practice). And just as they expect patients to heed the advice of their physicians, they should also follow "doctor's orders" in their own case.

Patients and providers have a common interest in creating a health care setting that provides the highest quality care. Such a setting might contain equal amounts of competence and trust; each depends, in part, on the other. Recommendations that would promote this common interest might thus have focused on the relationship between HCWs and patients. The CDC could have encouraged a conversation between patient and provider that would help tear down the blinds of suspicion and build the bonds of trust. The patient inquires and decides. The HCW advises and assures. This should make the health care setting healthier and more satisfying for both.

THE FINAL STEP

The final step in conflict resolution involves anticipating future conflict. This may be the most difficult step of all. The CDC officials, as well as just about everybody else involved in these issues, must be frustrated and exhausted that five full years after Bergalis was diagnosed with AIDS we have not yet arrived at a policy consensus regarding what to do about it.

But even now the time is ripe to address once again the issue of HIV in the health care workplace. Though the conflicts remain unresolved, we have had a long cooling-down period. The courts are now not as active; the states are no longer passing much legislation; Congress is working on other things; scholars are busy doing different research. Yet we now also have five additional years of experiments and analysis to help guide us.

It may be tempting to let this matter rest until another patient contracts HIV from a medical provider. But then it will be too late. We should act now to build consensus on appropriate public health policies, or we may well face another episode of bitterness, fear, and recriminations over a fatal extraction.

Appendix One

Forty-year-old white male in a general dentistry practice since 1980. Prior to that, he was in the military.

History of hepatitis B years ago.

Patient is bisexual. Went to a counseling and testing site some distance away (Ft. Lauderdale) from his residence in 1987 and was shocked to have been HIV positive. He was told that his immune system was intact at that time, but developed KS [Kaposi's sarcoma] in September 1987. He has also had an episode of presumptive PCP [pneumonia]. His physician is in Ft. Lauderdale and he received medical care at the Miami Veterans Administration Hospital.

He feels that he was infected through sexual activity, not occupationally. When his office is called, patients are told he has developed cancer, but he has heard that several people know that he has AIDS. His parents have moved from Pittsburgh to live with him.

He estimates that he had between 3,000 and 4,000 patients, and about 800–1,000 saw him every 6 months or so. He was one of the dentists on the state/county employees dental plan [CIGNA Dental Health]—that is why CDC#242284 [the CDC code for Bergalis] sought dental care from him. He estimates that he had about 10 persons in his practice who may have had HIV infection, and he was always "extra-careful" about infection control practices when he did procedures on these patients. He has worn gloves for patients he felt were "high risk" for years, but with the advent of HIV (can't remember exactly what year—thinks it was 1987)—he and hygienists always wore masks and new gloves for each patient. He did have an autoclave [heat sterilizer] but did not autoclave instruments after each patient. He did not recollect details of the infection control procedures, but said that prior to the mid 1980s they used alcohol to disinfect equipment, but after HIV switched to recommended "stronger disinfectants."

He does not recall any incident where he sustained a severe cut doing a procedure. He does recall occasionally being stuck recapping the narrow gauge needle used to administer anesthetic, but said that usually the assistant would be the one to be stuck as she recapped the needle.

He sold his practice in the summer of 1989, and his office files are not organized. He had only one filing box at home with a few of his patients' dental records (those who owed him money). The remainder of his files are scattered in many places—some are in his old office (he suspects that the new office has discarded some), patients who have gone to new dentists have picked theirs up, and those in the state/county dental plan are in another office. His books are also disorganized, and he did not appear to have a patient roster. He did not have his 1987 appointment book.

He has retained an attorney to deal with future interactions with CDC or the local health department.

We reviewed the dental records of CDC#242284 [Bergalis] with the dentist who took over the county health plan, who has never seen the patient. The teeth were not impacted and this was a simple extraction of the two upper wisdom teeth, which is [a] rather simple procedure requiring local anesthesia and dental extractors, which resemble pliers. He [this dentist] told us that there was no indication from the record that anything unusual had happened, and that in general, he had been impressed with the level of documentation in CDC#158093's [CDC code for Acer] charts.

Source: CDC, untitled interview notes on David Acer, n.d.

Appendix Two

━━ᠰᠣᠣ━━ Selected Bibliography Regarding Policies for
HIV-Positive Health Care Workers

Anderson, D. R. "Out for Blood: Mandatory AIDS Testing," *Maryland Bar
Journal 28* (May/June 1995), pp. 6–14.
Association for Practitioners in Infection Control and the Society of Hos-
pital Epidemiologists of America. "Position Paper: The HIV-Infected
Health Care Worker," *Infection Control and Hospital Epidemiology 11*
(1990), pp. 647–56.
Barnes, M., Rango, N. A., Burke, G. R., and Chiarello, L. "The HIV-Infected
Health Care Professional: Employment Policies and Public Health,"
Law, Medicine, and Health Care 18 (Winter 1990), pp. 311–30.
Brennan, T. A. "Transmission of the HIV in the Health Care Setting: Time
for Action," *New England Journal of Medicine 324* (May 23, 1991),
pp. 1504–7.
Cavender, J. W. "AIDS in the Health Care Setting: The Congressional
Response to the Kimberly Bergalis Case," *Georgia Law Review 26*
(1992), pp. 539–99.
Corless, I. B. "Much Ado About Something: The Restriction of HIV-
Infected Health-Care Providers," *AIDS and Public Policy Journal 7*
(Summer 1992), pp. 82–88.
Daniels, N. "HIV-Infected Health Care Professionals: Public Threat or Pub-
lic Sacrifice," *The Milbank Quarterly 70* (March 22, 1992), pp. 3–42.
Daniels, N. "HIV-Infected Professionals, Patient Rights, and the 'Switching
Dilemma,'" *Journal of the American Medical Association 267* (Mar. 11,
1992), pp. 1368–71.
Eisenstat, S. "The HIV-Infected Health Care Worker: The New AIDS Scape-
goat," *Rutgers Law Review 44* (1992) pp. 301–33.
Feldblum, C. "A Response to Gostin, 'The HIV-Infected Health Care Pro-
fessional: Public Policy, Discrimination, and Patient Safety,'" *Law,
Medicine, and Health Care 19* (1991), pp. 134–39.
Glantz, L. H., Mariner, W. K., and Annas, G. J. "Risky Business: Setting Pub-
lic Health Policy for HIV-Infected Health Care Professionals," *The
Milbank Quarterly 70* (March 22, 1992), pp. 43–79.

Gostin, L. "Hospitals, Health Care Professionals, and AIDS: The 'Right to Know' the Health Status of Professionals and Patients," *Maryland Law Review 48* (1989), pp. 12–54.

Gostin, L. "The HIV-Infected Health Care Professional: Public Policy, Discrimination, and Patient Safety," *Law, Medicine, and Health Care 18* (Winter 1990), pp. 303–10.

Johnson, J. A. "HIV-Infected Health Care Workers: The Medical and Scientific Issues," CRS Report no. 91–622 SPR (Nov. 15, 1991).

Jones, N. L. "HIV-Infected Health Care Workers: The Legal Issues," CRS Report no. 91–598A (Aug. 12, 1991).

Lieberman, K. C., and Derse, A. R. "HIV-Positive Health Care Workers and the Obligation to Disclose: Do Patients Have a Right to Know?," *Journal of Legal Medicine 13* (1992), pp. 333–56.

Lo, B., and Steinbrook, R. "HCWs Infected with the HIV," *Journal of the American Medical Association 267* (Feb. 26, 1992), pp. 1100–5.

Margolis, T. E. "Health Care Workers and AIDS: HIV Transmission in the Health Care Environment," *Journal of Legal Medicine 13* (1992), pp. 357–96.

U.S. Office of Technology Assessment. *HIV in the Health Care Workplace*, OTA-BP-H-90 (Nov. 1991).

Appendix Three

Organizations Represented at CDC Meetings Concerning Transmission of Bloodborne Pathogens to Patients During Invasive Procedures, August 1990 and February 1991

Note: Organizations attending the first meeting are denoted (1). Those speaking at the second meeting are denoted (2). Those attending the first meeting and speaking at the second are denoted (Both).

ACT-UP Atlanta (2)

AIDS Action Council (Both)

AIDS National Interfaith Network (2)

Alta Bates–Herrick Hospital (2)

American Academy of Family Physicians (1)

American Academy of Orthopaedic Surgeons (2)

American Academy of Pediatrics (Both)

American Association of Dental Schools (Both)

American Association of Occupational Health Nurses (2)

American Association of Oral Maxillofacial Surgeons (1)

American Association of Physicians for Human Rights (Both)

American Association of Public Health Dentistry (Both)

American Association of State and Territorial Dental Directors (Both)

American Civil Liberties Union AIDS Project (2)

American College of Emergency Physicians (Both)

American College of Obstetricians and Gynecologists (1)

American College of Physicians (Both)

American College of Surgeons (Both)

American Dental Association (Both)

American Dental Hygienists' Association (Both)

American Federation of State, County, and Municipal Employees (Both)

American Hospital Association (Both)

American Medical Association (Both)

American National Red Cross (2

American Nurses Association (Both)

American Occupational Health Nurses (1)

American Psychological Association (1)

American Public Health Association (Both)

American Society of Clinical Pathology (2)

American Society of Law and Medicine (Both)

Association for Practitioners in Infection Control; Society of Hospital
Epidemiologists of America (APIC/SHEA) HIV/AIDS Task Force (1)

Asian American Health Forum (1)

Association for Minority Health Professions Schools (1)

Association for Practitioners in Infection Control (1)

Association of American Medical Colleges (1)

Association of Operating Room Nurses (1)

Association of Practitioners in Infection Control (2)

Association of State and Territorial Dental Directors (Both)

Association of State and Territorial Health Officials (Both)

Association of the Bar of the City of New York (2)

Bay Area Physicians for Human Rights (2)

Bureau of Communicable Disease Epidemiology (1)

California AIDS Leadership Committee (2)

Canadian Dental Association (2)

College of American Pathologists (2)

Committee on Occupational AIDS (2)

Community Consortium in San Francisco (2)

Council of State and Territorial Epidemiologists (Both)

Drug, Hospital, and Health Care Employees Union (2)

Epidemiology and Infection Control (Canada)

Federation of Nurses and Health Professionals (2)

Florida Medical Association AIDS Activities (2)

Florida Department of Health and Rehabilitative Services (Both)

Florida House of Representatives (2)

French Ministry of Health (2)

Gay Men's Health Crisis (2)

Georgia AIDS Coalition (2)

Georgia Association of Physicians for Human Rights (2)

Harvard University Medical School (2)

The Hastings Center (1)

Human Rights Campaign Fund (2)

Infectious Disease Society of America (2)

International Association of Firefighters (1)

International Institute for Occupational Safety and Health (2)

Johns Hopkins University School of Hygiene and Public Health (2)

Johns Hopkins University School of Medicine (1)

Journal of the American Medical Association (2)

Lakeland Dental Center (2)

Lambda Legal Defense and Education Fund (2)

Local 1199 of the Retail, Wholesale, and Department Union (1)

Los Alamos National Laboratory (1)

Los Angeles County Department of Health (2)

Massachusetts Department of Health (1)

Medical College of Georgia (2)

Medical Expertise Retention Program (2)

Mercy Mobile Health Program (2)

Michigan State Department of Health (2)

Minnesota Department of Health (Both)

Mount Sinai Medical Center, New York (1)

National Association of County Health Officials (1)

National Association of Emergency Medical Technicians (1)

National Association of People Living with AIDS (2)

National Association of People with AIDS (1)

National Association of Social Workers (1)

National Coalition of Hispanic Health and Human Services Organizations (1)

National Commission on AIDS (2)

National Dental Association (1)

National Foundation for Infectious Diseases (2)

National Gay and Lesbian Task Force (2)

National Minority AIDS Council (2)

National Society for Patient Representation and Consumer Affairs (1)

New Jersey Medical School (2)

New York City Commission on Human Rights (2)

New York City Commission on Civil Rights (2)

New York City Health and Hospitals Corporation (2)

New York County Medical Society (2)

New York Department of Health (2)

New York Medical College (1)

New York Physicians for Human Rights (2)

New York State Department of Health (2)

New York State Division of Human Rights (2)

New York State Public Employees Federation (2)

North Carolina State Health Department (2)

Office of Sterilization and Asepsis Procedures Research Foundation (2)

Peekskill Area Health Center (2)

Rocky Mountain Infection Control Association (2)

San Francisco Health Commission (2)

Scientific Advisory Committee for the Community Consortium (2)

Service Employees International Union of the AFL-CIO (Both)

Society of Hospital Epidemiologists of America (Both)

Society of Thoracic Surgeons (1)

Surgical Infection Society (1)

U.S. Conference of City Health Officers (2)

U.S. Conference of Local Health Officials (Both)

United States Fire Administration (1)

University of California, San Francisco (2)

University of Florida (2)

University of Medicine and Dentistry of New Jersey (2)

University of Michigan School of Public Health (2)

University of Minnesota (1)

University of Texas Dental School (2)

University of Utah Medical School (2)

Vanderbilt University Hospital (1)

Vermont Diamond Instruments (2)

Washington University School of Medicine (1)

Yale University (2)

FEDERAL AGENCIES

Department of Veterans Affairs

Food and Drug Administration

National AIDS Program Office

National Cancer Institute, National Institutes of Health

National Institute of Dental Research, National Institutes of Health

National Institutes of Health

Occupational Safety and Health Administration

U.S. Air Force Surgeon General's Office

U.S. Army Surgeon General's Office

U.S. Navy Surgeon General's Office

Appendix Four

CDC Recommendations for Preventing Transmission of HIV and Hepatitis B Virus to Patients: Selected Sections

Infection Control

All HCWs *should* adhere to universal precautions, including the appropriate use of hand washing, protective barriers, and care in the use and disposal of needles and other sharp instruments. HCWs who have exudative lesions or weeping dermatitis *should* refrain from all direct patient care and from handling patient-care equipment and devices used in performing invasive procedures until the condition resolves. HCWs *should* also comply with current guidelines for disinfection and sterilization of reusable devices used in invasive procedures.

Practice Restrictions

Currently available data provide no basis for recommendations to restrict the practice of HCWs infected with HIV or HBVs who perform invasive procedures not identified as exposure-prone, provided the infected HCWs practice recommended surgical or dental technique and comply with universal precautions and current recommendations for sterilization/disinfection. Exposure-prone *should* be identified by medical, surgical, or dental organizations and institutions at which the procedures are performed.

HCWs who are infected with HIV or HBV *should not* perform exposure-prone procedures unless they have sought counsel from an expert review panel and been advised under what circumstances, if any, they may continue to perform these procedures.

HIV Testing

HCWs who perform exposure-prone procedures *should* know their HIV antibody status. . . . Mandatory testing of HCWs for HIV . . . is not recommended. The current assessment of the risk that infected

HCWs will transmit HIV or HBV to patients during exposure-prone procedures does not support the diversion of resources that would be required to implement mandatory testing programs. Compliance by HCWs with recommendations can be increased through education, training, and appropriate confidentiality safeguards.

Patient Notification

Such circumstances *would* include notifying prospective patients of the HCW's seropositivity before they undergo exposure-prone invasive procedures.

Note: Emphasis added.

Source: CDC, "Recommendations for Preventing Transmission of Human Immunodeficiency Virus and Hepatitis B Virus to Patients During Exposure-Prone Invasive Procedures," *MMWR 40* (July 12, 1991), pp. 5–6.

—ᴠᴠᴠ— Notes

Chapter One

1. L. K. Altman, "AIDS Mystery That Won't Go Away: Did a Dentist Infect Six Patients?" *New York Times*, July 5, 1994, p. B6.
2. The letter, dated April 6, 1991, originally appeared in the *Miami Herald*; it was reprinted as K. Bergalis, "I Blame Every One of You Bastards," reprinted in B. Kantrowitz, "Doctors with AIDS," *Newsweek*, July 1, 1991, p. 52.
3. The CDC initially reported the Bergalis case in "Possible Transmission of Human Immunodeficiency Virus to a Patient During an Invasive Dental Procedure," *Morbidity and Mortality Weekly Report* (hereafter *MMWR*) 30 (July 27, 1990), p. 491. All six cases were reported in CDC, "Update: Investigations of Persons Treated by HIV-Infected Health Care Workers—United States," *MMWR 42* (1993), pp. 329–31, 337.
4. CBS, *60 Minutes*, June 19, 1994; S. Barr, "What If the Dentist Didn't Do It?," *New York Times*, April 16, 1994, p. 21. Barr elaborated on these ideas in "In Defense of the AIDS Dentist," *Lear's*, April 1994, pp. 68–82. See also F. Rich, "The Gay Card," *New York Times*, June 26, 1994, p. D17.
5. C. A. Ciesielski and others, "The 1990 Florida Dental Investigation: The Press and the Science," *Annals of Internal Medicine 121* (Dec. 1, 1994), pp. 886–88.
6. G. Kolata, "The Face That Haunts," *New York Times*, July 10, 1994, p. D6.
7. G. E. Herbeck, "HIV and Dentistry," letter to the *Orlando Sentinel*, July 7, 1994, p. A12.
8. F. Rich, "The Gay Card," p. D17.
9. See especially C. A. Ciesielski and others, "Transmission of Human Immunodeficiency Virus in a Dental Practice," *Annals of Internal Medicine 116* (1992), pp. 798–805.
10. CBS, *60 Minutes*, June 19, 1994; Barr, "What If the Dentist Didn't Do It?," p. 21.
11. See, for example, BBC, *Panorama*, "AIDS Dental Mystery"; D. L. Lewis, letter responding to D. L. Breo, "The Dental AIDS Cases: Murder or Unsolvable Mystery?" *JAMA 271* (1994), p. 983.

12. For example, U.S. General Accounting Office, *AIDS: CDC's Investigation of HIV Transmissions by a Dentist* (Washington, D.C.: U.S. GAO, 1992); R. Runnells, *AIDS in the Dental Office? The Story of Kimberly Bergalis and Dr. David Acer* (Fruit Heights, Utah: IC Publications, 1993).

13. ABC, *20/20,* "Was it Murder?," Oct. 1, 1993; MoPo Productions, Paramount Domestic Television, *Maury Povich Show,* "Dr. Acer's Young Victim," Sept. 15, 1993. See also, for example, D. R. Pepper, letter responding to Breo, "The Dental AIDS Cases," p. 983; Leonard G. Horowitz, *Deadly Innocence: Solving the Greatest Murder Mystery in the History of American Medicine* (Rockport, Mass.: Tetrahedron Industries, 1994).

14. Koop statement to journalists, Lansing, Mich., March 1993.

15. CDC, "Recommendations for Preventing Transmission of HIV in Health-Care Settings," *MMWR 36* (1987), p. 305.

16. Reported in Kantrowitz, "Doctors with AIDS," p. 51.

17. E. W. Etheridge, *Sentinel for Health: A History of the Centers for Disease Control* (Berkeley: University of California Press, 1992).

18. S. Panem, *The AIDS Bureaucracy* (Cambridge, Mass.: Harvard University Press, 1988), pp. 40–43.

19. First reported in CDC, "Respiratory Infection—Pennsylvania," *MMWR 25* (1976), p. 244; resolved in CDC, "Follow-up on Respiratory Illness—Philadelphia," *MMWR 26* (1977), pp. 9–11. See also Committee on Human Resources, U.S. Senate, *Follow-up Examination on Legionnaires' Disease,* hearing before the Subcommittee on Health and Scientific Research, 95th Congress, Nov. 9, 1977 (Washington, D.C.: U.S. Government Printing Office, 1977). For a discussion, see G. L. Lattimer and R. A. Ormsbee, *Legionnaires' Disease* (New York: Marcel Dekker, 1981).

20. R. Shilts, *And the Band Played On: Politics, People, and the AIDS Epidemic* (New York: St. Martin's Press, 1987).

21. CDC, "*Pneumocystis Pneumonia*—Los Angeles," *MMWR 30* (June 5, 1981), pp. 250–51.

22. CDC, "Kaposi's Sarcoma and *Pneumocystis Pneumonia* Among Homosexual Men—New York City and California," *MMWR 30* (July 3, 1981), pp. 305–7.

23. Etheridge, *Sentinel for Health,* p. 324.

24. CDC, "*Pneumocystis Carinii* Pneumonia Among Persons with Hemophilia A," *MMWR 31* (July 16, 1982), pp. 365–67.

25. R. Bayer, *Private Acts and Social Consequences* (New York: Free Press, 1989), pp. 72–100; and Etheridge, *Sentinel for Health,* pp. 330–37.

26. Etheridge, *Sentinel for Health,* p. 333.

27. Etheridge, *Sentinel for Health,* p. 333.

28. B. Evatt, quoted in Etheridge, *Sentinel for Health,* p. 334.

29. Etheridge, *Sentinel for Health*, p. 334.

30. In particular, Ciesielski and others, "The 1990 Florida Dental Investigation"; Ciesielski and others, "Transmission of Human Immunodeficiency Virus in a Dental Practice."

31. J. Q. Wilson, *Bureaucracy: What Government Agencies Do and Why They Do It* (New York: Basic Books, 1989).

32. R. A. Katzmann, *Regulatory Bureaucracy: The Federal Trade Commission and Antitrust Policy* (Cambridge, Mass.: MIT Press, 1980).

33. M. C. Rom, *Public Spirit in the Thrift Tragedy* (Pittsburgh, Pa.: University of Pittsburgh Press, 1996).

34. Interview with S. Kuvin, Nov. 7, 1995.

35. D. P. Francis, "Toward a Comprehensive HIV Prevention Program for the CDC and the Nation," *JAMA 268* (Sept. 16, 1992), pp. 1444–47; 1445.

36. R. Kerrison, "Innocent Girl's Blood on Politicians' Hands," *Human Events*, reprinted in *Congressional Record*, July 18, 1991, p. S10340.

Chapter Two

1. Interview with C. Ciesielski, Dec. 18, 1991.

2. CDC, *HIV/AIDS Surveillance Report* (Washington, D.C.: CDC, 1991), p. 10.

3. CDC, *HIV/AIDS Surveillance Report*, p. 10.

4. CDC, *HIV/AIDS Surveillance Report*, p. 10.

5. See, for example, Special Initiative on AIDS, "Contact Tracing and Partner Notification" (Washington, D.C.: American Public Health Association, 1988).

6. M. L. Norris, "Tracking the Path of AIDS," *Washington Post*, May 31, 1992, p. A1.

7. Norris, "Tracking the Path of AIDS," p. A20.

8. Data on male bisexuality in the United States are rare. See L. S. Doll, J. Peterson, J. R. Magana, and J. M. Carrier, "Male Bisexuality and AIDS in the United States," in *Bisexuality and HIV/AIDS: A Global Perspective* (Amherst, N.Y.: Prometheus Books, 1991), pp. 27–40.

9. Interview with N. Economou, Jan. 8, 1992.

10. A. Hull, "AIDS and the Student Body," *St. Petersburg Times*, Jan. 18, 1987, p. 1F.

11. Interview with Economou, Jan. 8, 1992.

12. Economou case report on Bergalis, Dec. 14, 1989, p. 18.

13. National Research Council, *Risking the Future: Adolescent Sexuality, Pregnancy, and Childbearing* (Washington, D.C.: National Academy Press, 1987).

14. M. Schuster, "The Sexual Practices of Adolescent Virgins," paper presented at the Robert Wood Johnson Foundation Clinical Scholars Program Annual Meeting, Ft. Lauderdale, Fla., Nov. 8–11, 1995.

15. Runnells, *AIDS in the Dental Office?*, p. 86.

16. CDC, *HIV/AIDS Surveillance Report*, p. 17.

17. Interview with Economou, Jan. 9, 1992.

18. CDC, *Guidelines for Reporting Epidemiological Investigations (EPI-AIDS)* (Washington, D.C.: CDC, n.d.).

19. CDC interview summaries, n.d.

20. "GAO Review of Dental Case Supports the CDC's Conclusions," *AIDS Alert 7* (Dec. 1992), pp. 183–85; quote on p. 184.

21. Ciesielski and others, "Transmission of Human Immunodeficiency Virus in a Dental Practice," pp. 798–805.

22. Ciesielski, untitled interview notes with D. Acer, n.d.

23. CDC notes on Bergalis medical records, March 28, 1988; this note is from Bergalis's college infirmary records, Oct. 20, 1987.

24. CDC notes on Bergalis medical records, March 28, 1988; this quote is from Bergalis's college infirmary records, Jan. 9, 1988.

25. CDC interview summaries, n.d.

26. CDC interview summaries, n.d.

27. Runnells, *AIDS in the Dental Office?*, pp. 89–90.

28. CDC interview summaries, n.d.

29. W. T. Gormley Jr., *Taming the Bureaucracy: Muscles, Prayers, and Other Strategies* (Princeton, N.J.: Princeton University Press, 1989).

30. E. Bardach and R. A. Kagan, *Going by the Book: The Problem of Regulatory Unreasonableness* (Philadelphia: Temple University Press, 1982).

31. D. E. Osborne and T. Gaebler, *Reinventing Government: How the Entrepreneurial Spirit Is Transforming the Public Sector* (Reading, Mass.: Addison-Wesley, 1992).

32. Deposition of K. Bergalis, for *Kimberly Bergalis v. David Acer*, Oct. 11, 1990, pp. 26–27.

33. Interview with G. and A. Bergalis, Jan. 9, 1996.

34. CBS, *60 Minutes*, June 19, 1994; S. Barr, "What If the Dentist Didn't Do It?" p. 21; Barr, "In Defense of the AIDS Dentist," pp. 68–82.

35. Barr, "In Defense of the AIDS Dentist," p. 69.

36. Ciesielski and others, "The 1990 Florida Dental Investigation," pp. 886–88.

37. Runnells, *AIDS in the Dental Office?*, pp. 105–9.

38. Barr, "In Defense of the AIDS Dentist," p. 79.

39. Barr, "In Defense of the AIDS Dentist," p. 79.

40. Letter from Witte and Miller to Curran, July 23, 1990.

41. CDC, "Possible Transmission," pp. 489–92.

42. CDC, "Possible Transmission," p. 491.

43. All quotes from CDC, "Possible Transmission," p. 491.

44. K. Bergalis, "Deposition," p. 30.

45. CDC, "Briefing Notes on *MMWR* Article, July 27, 1990," (July 25, 1990). The briefing notes were distributed through a memo from Jaffe.

46. The 1987 citation comes from CDC, "Recommendations for Prevention of HIV Transmission in Health-Care Settings," *MMWR* (Aug. 21, 1987).

47. CDC, "Briefing Notes."

48. Dated Aug. 24, 1990.

49. Florida State Section 455.241; see "Authorization for Release."

50. Florida Statute Chapter 384; see "Authorization for Release."

51. HRS, unlabeled draft, Aug. 8, 1990.

52. This section is based on Ciesielski and others, "Transmission of Human Immunodeficiency Virus in a Dental Practice," pp. 798–805; Ciesielski and others, "The 1990 Florida Dental Investigation," pp. 886–88; CDC case records obtained from Robert Montgomery of Montgomery and Larmoyeux; and various newspaper reports.

53. Barr, "In Defense of the AIDS Dentist," p. 81.

Chapter Three

1. G. Myers and others, "Human Retroviruses and AIDS, 1989" (Los Alamos, N.M.: Los Alamos National Laboratory, Theoretical Division, 1989).

2. R. C. Bohinski, *Modern Concepts in Biochemistry,* 3rd ed. (Needham Heights, Mass.: Allyn & Bacon, 1979), p. 204.

3. C.-Y. Ou and others, "Molecular Epidemiology of HIV Transmission in a Dental Practice," *Science 256* (1992), pp. 1165–71; C. L. Kuiken and B. Korber, "Epidemiological Significance of Intra- and Inter-person Variation in HIV–1," *AIDS 8,* suppl. 1 (1994), pp. S73–S83.

4. G. Myers, personal correspondence with author, Nov. 8, 1996.

5. See also GAO, *AIDS: CDC's Investigation,* p. 23, which identifies the first four stages.

6. CDC, "Possible Transmission of HIV to a Patient," p. 492.

7. CDC, "Update: Transmission of HIV Infection During an Invasive Dental Procedure—Florida," *MMWR 40* (Jan. 18, 1991), pp. 21–27, 33.

8. CDC, "Update: Transmission of HIV Infection During an Invasive Dental Procedure—Florida," *MMWR 40* (June 14, 1991), pp. 377–81.

9. Ou and others, "Molecular Epidemiology," pp. 1165–71, marked the end of this stage.

10. CDC, "Update: Investigations of Persons Treated by HIV-Infected Health-Care Workers—United States," *MMWR 42* (May 7, 1993), pp. 329–30.

11. C.-Y. Ou and others, "DNA Amplification for Direct Detection of HIV–1 in DNA of Peripheral Blood Mononuclear Cells," *Science 238* (1988), pp. 295–97.

12. M. A. Innis, D. H. Gelfand, J. J. Sninsky, and T. J. White, eds., *PCR Protocols: A Guide to Methods and Applications* (New York: Academic Press, 1990), pp. xvii–xviii.

13. D. Kellog and S. Kwok, "Detection of Human Immunodeficiency Virus," in Innis, Gelfand, Sninsky, and White, *PCR Protocols*, p. 338.

14. Ou and others, "Molecular Epidemiology," fn. 15 and 17, p. 1170.

15. J. Cohen, "Unlikely Recruit: Andrew Leigh Brown, Population Geneticist, Studies HIV Transmission," *Science 260* (May 28, 1993), p. 1264.

16. Fax from A. Leigh Brown to C.-Y. Ou, n.d.

17. J. Palca, "Trying to Pin Down an Ever-Changing Virus," *Science 255* (Jan. 24, 1992), p. 393.

18. See J. Palca, "CDC Closes the Case of the Florida Dentist," *Science 256* (May 22, 1992), pp. 1130–31; T. F. Smith and M. S. Waterman, "The Continuing Case of the Florida Dentist," *Science 256* (May 22, 1992), pp. 1155–56.

19. D. Rosenthal, *At the Heart of the Bomb: The Dangerous Allure of Weapons Work* (Reading, Mass.: Addison-Wesley, 1990).

20. J. D. Watson, "The Human Genome Project: Past, Present, and Future," *Science 248* (Apr. 6, 1990), pp. 44ff.

21. Myers, personal correspondence with author, Nov. 8, 1996.

22. J. Crewdson, "In Gallo Case, Truth Termed a Casualty: Science Subverted in AIDS Dispute," *Chicago Tribune*, Jan. 1, 1995, p. 1.

23. "Molecular Epidemiology of AIDS," Interagency agreement among the Centers for Disease Control, National Center for Infectious Diseases, and the Department of Energy, Los Alamos National Laboratory, Aug. 14, 1991.

24. Myers, personal correspondence with author, Nov. 7, 1996.

25. Myers speaks at greatest length about his research in "The Oral and Video-taped Deposition of Dr. Gerald Myers," *Richard L. Driskill* v. *CIGNA Dental Health of Florida, Inc.*, 19th Judicial Circuit Court of Florida, Apr. 24, 1991.

26. Interview with Myers, Atlanta, Jan. 29, 1992.

27. Fax from Myers to Jaffe and Ciesielski, July 24, 1990.

28. Fax from Myers to Jaffe and Ciesielski, July 24, 1990.

29. Myers's emphasis. Fax from Myers to Jaffe and Ciesielski, July 24, 1990.

30. J. I. Mullins, unpublished letter, July 26, 1990.

31. Emphasis added. CDC, "Possible Transmission," p. 491.

32. CDC, "Possible Transmission," p. 491.

33. CDC, "Update: Transmission of HIV Infection," *MMWR 40* (Jan. 18, 1991), p. 25.

34. See, for example, R. Higgs, *Crisis and Leviathan: Critical Episodes in the*

Growth of American Government (New York: Oxford University Press, 1987); and J. T. Bennett and T. J. DiLorenzo, *Official Lies: How Washington Misleads Us* (Alexandria, Va.: Groom Books, 1992).

35. G. Taubes, "Epidemiology Faces Its Limits," *Science 269* (July 14, 1995), pp. 164–69. See also C. B. Begg and J. A. Berlin, "Publication Bias: A Problem in Interpreting Medical Data," *Journal of the Royal Statistical Society 151*, series A, (1988), pp. 1–27; and R. Rosenthal, "The 'File Drawer Problem' and Tolerance for Null Results," *Psychological Bulletin 86* (1978), pp. 638–41.

36. L. Day, *AIDS: What the Government Isn't Telling You* (Palm Desert, Calif.: Rockford Press, 1991).

37. See D. M. Hillis, J. P. Huelsenbeck, and C. W. Cunningham, "Application and Accuracy of Molecular Phylogenies," *Science 264* (Apr. 29, 1994), pp. 671–77; and Hillis and Huelsenbeck, "Support for Dental HIV Transmission," letter to *Nature 369* (May 5, 1994), pp. 24–25. A critique of Myers's analysis was published as a letter by R. W. DeBry and others, "Dental HIV Transmission," *Nature 361* (Feb. 25, 1993), p. 691. For a discussion of the scientific controversies, see Palca, "The Case of the Florida Dentist," *Science 255* (Jan. 24, 1992), pp. 392–94, and Palca, "CDC Closes the Case of the Florida Dentist," pp. 1130–31.

38. Interview with Myers, Jan. 29, 1992.

39. CDC, "Possible Transmission," p. 490.

40. G. Myers and others (eds.), "Human Retroviruses and AIDS 1991: A Compilation and Analysis of Nucleic Acid and Amino Acid Sequences" (Los Alamos, N.M.: Los Alamos National Laboratory, Theoretical Division, T10, 1991).

41. CDC, "Epidemiologic Study of the DNA Sequencing Technique to Clarify the Mode of Transmission of HIV in an AIDS Patient with No Identified Risk," Protocol no. 980, June 26, 1990.

42. CDC, "Comparisons of Sequencing Data," unpublished, no date.

43. Myers, "Deposition of Dr. Gerald Myers," pp. 71–76.

44. Interview with Korber, Aug. 4, 1994.

45. Korber and Myers, "Signature Pattern Analysis," pp. 1549–60.

46. Mullins, unpublished letter, July 26, 1990.

47. Ou and others, "Molecular Epidemiology," p. 1168.

Chapter Four

1. B. Gooch and others, "Lack of Evidence for Patient-to-Patient Transmission of HIV in a Dental Practice," *Journal of the American Dental Association 124* (Jan. 1993), pp. 38–44.

2. Interview with Marianos and Gooch, Dec. 12, 1991.

3. Ciesielski and others, "Transmission of HIV in a Dental Practice," pp. 803–804.

4. CDC, "Estimates of the Risk of Endemic Transmission of HBV and HIV to Patients by the Percutaneous Route During Invasive Surgical and Dental Procedures," unpublished draft, Jan. 30, 1991, p. 3. "Percutaneous" means passing through unbroken skin. *Stedman's Medical Dictionary: Lawyers' Edition*, 5th ed. (Baltimore: Williams and Wilkins, 1982), p. 1052.

5. Abel, Miller, Mecik, and Ryge, "Studies on Dental Aerobiology, IV," pp. 1567–69; and M. V. Martin, "The Significance of the Bacterial Contamination of Dental Unit Water Systems," *British Journal of Dentistry 163* (1987), pp. 152–54.

6. CDC, "Estimates of the Risk," p. 3.

7. D. L. Lewis and R. K. Boe, "Cross-Infection Risks Associated with Current Procedures for Using High-Speed Dental Handpieces," *Journal of Clinical Microbiology 30* (Feb. 1992), pp. 401–6; D. L. Lewis and others, "Cross-Contamination Potential with Dental Equipment," *The Lancet 340* (Nov. 21, 1992), pp. 1252–54.

8. Lewis and others, "Cross-Contamination," p. 1253.

9. G. J. Christensen, "Infection Control: Some Significant Loopholes," *Journal of the American Dental Association 122* (Aug. 1991), pp. 99–100.

10. Christensen, "Infection Control," p. 100.

11. C. Russell, "Dental Drills and the Risk of Infection: Methods of Disinfecting Instruments Between Patients Raise Concern," *Washington Post*, Jan. 28, 1992, Health section, pp. 6–7.

12. Runnells, *AIDS in the Dental Office?*, p. 58.

13. CDC, "Update: Transmission of HIV Infection," Jan. 18, 1991, pp. 21–27, 33; and Ciesielski and others, "Transmission of Human Immunodeficiency Virus in a Dental Practice," pp. 798–805.

14. Ciesielski and others, "Transmission of Human Immunodeficiency Virus in a Dental Practice," p. 802.

15. Gooch and others, "Lack of Evidence for Patient-to-Patient Transmission," p. 38.

16. See CDC, "Recommendations for Prevention of HIV Transmission in Health-Care Settings," *MMWR 36* (supplement 25) (1987), p. 7S.

17. GAO, *AIDS: CDC's Investigation*, p. 44.

18. Deposition of Elizabeth Greenhill, D.D.S., in *Driskill v. CIGNA*, May 28, 1991, pp. 10–11.

19. Greenhill deposition, pp. 10–11.

20. Deposition of Margaret D. Crawford, *Bergalis* v. *CIGNA*, March 26, 1991, p. 8.
21. Runnells, *AIDS in the Dental Office?*, p. 256.
22. Deposition of Diane Rubeck, *Driskill* v. *CIGNA*, April 15, 1992, pp. 9, 13.
23. Runnells, *AIDS in the Dental Office?*, p. 261.
24. CDC, "Update: Investigations of Persons Treated by HIV-Infected Health-Care Workers," p. 330.
25. Ciesielski and others, "Transmission of Human Immunodeficiency Virus in a Dental Practice," p. 802.
26. Crawford deposition, March 26, 1991.
27. Ciesielski and others, "Transmission of Human Immunodeficiency Virus in a Dental Practice," p. 802.
28. D. K. Henderson and others, "Risk of Occupational Transmission of Human Immunodeficiency Virus Type 1 (HIV–1) Associated with Clinical Exposures: A Prospective Evaluation," *Annals of Internal Medicine 113* (1990), pp. 740–46; R. Marcus and the CDC Cooperative Needlestick Study Group, "Surveillance of Health-Care Workers Exposed to Blood from Patients Infected with the Human Immunodeficiency Virus," *New England Journal of Medicine 319* (1988), pp. 1118–23; M. E. Chamberland and others, "Health Care Workers with AIDS: National Surveillance Update," *Journal of the American Medical Association 266* (1991), pp. 3459–62.
29. N. M. Flynn and others, "Absence of HIV Antibody Among Dental Professionals Exposed to Infected Patients," *Western Journal of Medicine 146* (1987), pp. 439–42.
30. R. S. Klein and others, "Low Occupational Risk of Human Immunodeficiency Virus Infection Among Dental Professionals," *New England Journal of Medicine 318* (1988), pp. 86–90.
31. See, for example, R. G. Miller, D. D. Kiprov, G. Parry, and D. E. Bredesen, "Peripheral Nervous System Dysfunction in Acquired Immunodeficiency Syndrome," in University of California School of Medicine, San Francisco, *AIDS and the Nervous System* (New York: Raven Press, 1988), pp. 65–78.
32. D. D. Ho, T. Moudgil, and M. Alam, "Quantitation of Human Immunodeficiency Virus Type 1 in the Blood of Infected Persons," *New England Journal of Medicine 321* (Dec. 14, 1989), pp. 1621–25.
33. G. Kolata, "For Heterosexuals, Diagnosis of AIDS Is Often Unmercifully Late," *New York Times*, Nov. 9, 1991, p. 32.
34. Ciesielski interview with Acer, March 29, 1990.
35. Ciesielski and others, "Transmission of Human Immunodeficiency Virus in a Dental Practice"; CDC, "Interview Questions for Dental Staff Members," unpublished, Sept. 1990.

36. Ciesielski and others, "Transmission of Human Immunodeficiency Virus in a Dental Practice," p. 801.

37. Runnells, *AIDS in the Dental Office?*, p. 75.

38. CDC, "Update: Investigations of Persons Treated by HIV-Infected Health-Care Workers," p. 330.

39. Public Citizen's Health Research Group, "Comparing State Medical Boards," 1992, summarized in *Health Law Reporter 2* (1993), pp. 73ff., and cited in A. S. Oddi, "Reverse Informed Consent: The Unreasonably Dangerous Patient," *Vanderbilt Law Review 46* (Nov. 1993), pp. 1417–76.

40. L. G. Horowitz, *Deadly Innocence* (Rockport, Mass.: Tetrahedron Industries, 1993); see also L. Altman, "AIDS and a Dentist's Secrets: Was It Murder?," *New York Times,* June 6, 1993, Sect. 4, p. 1.

41. R. Hiaasen, "Friend Believes Acer Meant to Transmit AIDS," *Palm Beach Post,* June 10, 1992, p. 1Aff.

42. Parsons made these statements in a Barbara Walters special on the CBS show *20/20.*

43. Deposition of Edward Parsons, in *Driskill* v. *CIGNA,* Jan. 2, 1992.

44. See D. J. Sears, *To Kill Again: The Motivation and Development of Serial Murder* (Wilmington, Del.: SR Books, 1991); and S. A. Egger, ed., *Serial Murder: An Elusive Phenomenon* (New York: Praeger Press, 1990).

45. Runnells, *AIDS in the Dental Office?*, p. 20.

46. Deposition of A. Bergalis, *Webb* v. *CIGNA* and *Driskill* v. *CIGNA,* April 26, 1991, pp. 19, 17.

47. Runnells, *AIDS in the Dental Office?*, p. 295.

48. Runnells, *AIDS in the Dental Office?*, p. 59.

49. Deposition of Parsons, Jan. 2, 1992.

50. Runnells, *AIDS in the Dental Office?*, p. 76.

51. Runnells, *AIDS in the Dental Office?*, p. 80.

52. F. L. Ford, *Political Murder: From Tyrannicide to Terrorism* (Cambridge, Mass.: Harvard University Press, 1985); and S. Anzovin, ed., *Terrorism* (New York: Wilson, 1986).

53. See, especially, Shilts, *And the Band Played On* and Panem, *The AIDS Bureaucracy.*

54. E. Kübler-Ross, *On Death and Dying* (New York: Macmillan, 1969); and Kübler-Ross, *AIDS: The Ultimate Challenge* (New York: Macmillan 1987).

55. Breo, "The Dental AIDS Cases: Murder or Unsolvable Mystery?" *JAMA 270* (Dec. 8, 1993), p. 2734.

56. For example, Breo, "The Dental AIDS Cases," p. 2732.

57. Breo, "The Dental AIDS Cases," pp. 2732, 2734.

58. Jaffe, quoted in L. K. Altman, "AIDS Mystery That Won't Go Away," p. B6.

Chapter Five

1. Runnells, *AIDS in the Dental Office?*, p. 143.
2. K. Bergalis, "I Blame Every One of You Bastards," p. 52.
3. A. Japenga, "The Secret," *Health*, Sept. 1992, p. 44.
4. *New York Times*, Feb. 9, 1991, p. 1A.
5. "New AHA Guidelines Urge Universal AIDS Precautions," *Medical Staff News 16* (Aug. 1987), p. 2.
6. Reported in Kantrowitz, "Doctors with AIDS," p. 51.
7. A history of proposals for mandatory HIV testing is contained in R. Bayer, *Private Acts, Social Consequences: AIDS and the Politics of Public Health* (New York: Free Press, 1989), pp. 137–68.
8. W. E. Chavey and others, "Cost-Effectiveness Analysis of Screening Health Care Workers for HIV," *Journal of Family Practice 38* (March 1994), pp. 249ff.
9. See C. R. Sunstein, *After the Rights Revolution: Reconceiving the Regulatory State* (Cambridge, Mass.: Harvard University Press, 1990), Appendix B, for the estimated cost per saved life of various regulations.
10. See D. R. Anderson, "Out for Blood: Mandatory AIDS Testing," *Maryland Bar Journal 28* (May–June 1995), pp. 6–14, for a discussion of the constitutional issues.
11. L. Gostin, "The HIV-Infected Health Care Professional: Public Policy, Discrimination, and Patient Safety," *Law, Medicine, and Health Care 18* (Winter 1990), pp. 303–10; quote on p. 307.
12. Gostin, "The HIV-Infected Health Care Professional," pp. 303–10.
13. Gostin, "The HIV-Infected Health Care Professional," p. 305.
14. M. Barnes, N. A. Rango, G. R. Burke, and L. Chiarello, "The HIV-Infected Health Care Professional: Employment Policies and Public Health," *Law, Medicine, and Health Care 18* (Winter 1990), pp. 311–30.
15. Authors' emphasis. Section 504; 29 U.S.C.A. sections 794.
16. *Prewitt* v. *U.S. Postal Service*, 662 F.2d 292, 306–07 (5th Cir. 1980).
17. 480 U.S. 273 (1987).
18. C. Marsh, Nassau County superintendent of schools, quoted in *Nassau County* v. *Arline*, 480 U.S. 273 (1987).
19. *Nassau County* v. *Arline*, p. 3.
20. Emphasis added. *Nassau County* v. *Arline*, pp. 3–4.
21. *Nassau County* v. *Arline*, p. 17.
22. "Americans with Disabilities Act of 1989, Hearing on S. 933 Before the Senate Committee on Labor and Human Resources and the Senate Subcommittee on the Handicapped," 101st Cong., 1st Sess. (Washington, D.C.: U.S. GPO, 1989), p. 616. For a recent case finding HIV infection a covered

disability under the Americans with Disabilities Act, see *Doe* v. *Kohn, Nast & Graf,* No. Civ. A. 93–4510, 1994 WL 416269 (E.D. Pa. 4 Aug. 1994).

23. For a discussion, see P. L. Gordon, "The Job Application Process after the Americans with Disabilities Act," *Employee Relations Law Journal 8* (Sept. 22, 1992), pp. 85ff.

24. Gordon, "The Job Application Process."

25. Gordon, "The Job Application Process."

26. Gostin, "The HIV-Infected Health Care Professional," p. 304.

27. Deposition of K. Bergalis, *Webb* v. *CIGNA,* 19th Judicial Circuit Court, Martin County, Case No. 91–280, CA, pp. 37–38 (Apr. 15, 1991).

28. Deposition of K. Bergalis, *Webb* v. *CIGNA,* pp. 37–38.

29. In Japenga, "The Secret," pp. 49, 52.

30. Gostin, "The HIV-Infected Health Care Professional," p. 304.

31. CDC, "Estimates of the Risk."

32. CDC, "Estimates of the Risk," p. 2.

33. J. I. Tokars and others, "Blood Contacts During Surgical Procedures," 30th Interscience Conference on Antimicrobial Agents and Chemotherapy, Abstract 958 (1990), p. 246.

34. See CDC, "Estimates of the Risk," pp. 6–7.

35. See CDC, "Estimates of the Risk," p. 4.

36. See CDC, "Estimates of the Risk," pp. 2–4.

37. CDC, "Estimates of the Risk," Table 4. See also L. Bernard and R. Steinbrook, "HCPs Infected with the HIV," *JAMA 267* (Feb. 26, 1992), pp. 1100–5.

38. N. Daniels, "HIV-Infected Health Care Professionals: Public Threat or Public Sacrifice," *The Milbank Quarterly 70* (March 22, 1992), pp. 3–42.

39. J. Hastings, "The Chances You Take," *Health* (Sept. 1992), p. 50.

40. Emphasis added. American Medical Association, Council on Ethical and Judicial Affairs, "Ethical Issues Involved in the Growing AIDS Crisis," *JAMA 259* (March 4, 1988), p. 361.

41. Emphasis added. American Medical Association, *Statement on HIV-Infected Physicians* (Jan. 17, 1991).

42. Barnes, Rango, Burke, and Chiarello, "The HIV-Infected Health Care Professional," pp. 314–15.

Chapter Six

1. CDC, "Acquired Immunodeficiency Syndrome (AIDS): Precautions for Clinical and Laboratory Staffs," *MMWR 31* (1982), pp. 577–80; CDC, "Acquired Immunodeficiency Syndrome (AIDS: Precautions for Health

Care Workers and Allied Professionals," *MMWR 32* (1983), pp. 450–51; CDC, "Recommendations for Preventing Transmission of Infection with Human T-lymphotropic Virus Type III/Lymphadenopathy-Associated Virus in the Workplace," *MMWR 34* (1985), pp. 681–86, 691–95; CDC, "Recommendations for Preventing Transmission of Infection with Human T-lymphotropic Virus Type III/Lymphadenopathy-Associated Virus During Invasive Procedures," *MMWR 35* (1986), pp. 221–23; CDC, "Recommendations for Prevention of HIV Transmission in Health-Care Settings," *MMWR 36,* suppl. no. 2S (1987), pp. 1–18S; CDC, "Update: Universal Precautions for Prevention of Transmission of Human Immunodeficiency Virus, Hepatitis B Virus, and Other Bloodborne Pathogens in Health-Care Settings," *MMWR 37* (1988), pp. 377–82, 387–88; CDC, "Guidelines for Prevention of Transmission of Human Immunodeficiency Virus and Hepatitis B Virus to Health-Care and Public-Safety Workers," *MMWR 38,* suppl. no. S6 (1989), pp. 1–37. As a shorthand, I will refer to these as, for example, the "1989 recommendations."

2. CDC, "Estimates of the Risk," p. 4.

3. On this point, see especially Barnes, Rango, Burke, and Chiarello, "The HIV-Infected Health Care Professional," pp. 311–30.

4. CDC, 1985 recommendations.

5. CDC, 1985 recommendations.

6. CDC, "Recommendations for Preventing Transmission of Human Immunodeficiency Virus and Hepatitis B Virus to Patients During Exposure-Prone Invasive Procedures," *MMWR 40* (July 12, 1991), henceforth "1991 recommendations."

7. CDC, 1986 recommendations, p. 221.

8. CDC, 1987 recommendations, p. 15S.

9. CDC, 1987 recommendations, p. 15S.

10. CDC, 1987 recommendations, p. 15S.

11. CDC, 1987 recommendations, p. 16S.

12. For a sustained discussion of bureaucratic rule making and the Administrative Procedures Act, see C. M. Kerwin, *Rulemaking: How Government Agencies Write Law and Make Policy* (Washington, D.C.: CQ Press, 1994).

13. Kerwin, *Rulemaking,* pp. 51–52.

14. Breo, "The Dental AIDS Cases," pp. 2733–34.

15. B. Mullan, "Centers for Disease Control Consultants Meeting: Prevention of Transmission of Bloodborne Pathogens to Patients During Invasive Procedures," personal notes, Aug. 13–14, 1990.

16. The classic study is S. Verba and N. H. Nie, *Participation in America: Political Participation and Social Equality* (New York: HarperCollins, 1972). The seminal work regarding the influence of organized interests over public

policy is G. McConnell, *Private Power and American Democracy* (New York: Vintage Books, 1966).

17. See Gormley, *Taming the Bureaucracy,* esp. chap. 3.

18. Mullan, "Consultants Meeting," p. 4.

19. Mullan, "Consultants Meeting," p. 22.

20. Mullan, "Consultants Meeting," p. 27.

21. Mullan, "Consultants Meeting," p. 30.

22. Breo, "The Dental AIDS Cases," p. 2734.

23. S. Sternberg, unpublished interview notes, July 17, 1992.

24. Comments by W. Roper, in CDC, "Open Meeting on the Risks of Transmission of Bloodborne Pathogens to Patients During Invasive Procedures" (Atlanta: CDC, Feb. 21–22, 1991), p. 3.

25. CDC, Notice of "Open Meeting on the Risks of Transmission of Bloodborne Pathogens to Patients During Invasive Procedures," *Federal Register* 56 (Jan. 23, 1991), p. 2527.

26. Comments by Roper, in CDC, "Open Meeting," pp. 4–5.

27. CDC, "Open Meeting," p. 49.

28. CDC, "Open Meeting," p. 52.

29. CDC, "Open Meeting," p. 97.

30. CDC, "Open Meeting," p. 69.

31. For example, see Bell comments, in CDC, "Open Meeting," pp. 62, 67.

32. CDC, "Open Meeting," p. 69.

33. Bell comments, in CDC, "Open Meeting," p. 47.

34. CDC, "Open Meeting," p. 87.

35. Roper comments, in CDC, "Open Meeting," p. 488.

36. Sternberg, notes, July 17, 1991.

37. CDC, "Draft Recommendations to Prevent Transmission of HIV and HBV from Health-Care Workers to Patients During Invasive Procedures," unpublished (March 25, 1991), p. 4.

38. W. L. Roper, "Draft Recommendations to Prevent Transmission of HIV and HBV from Health-Care Workers to Patients During Invasive Procedures— ACTION," Apr. 5, 1991, p. 6.

39. CDC, "Draft Recommendations," p. 6.

40. Roper, "Draft Recommendations," p. 9.

41. Roper, "Draft Recommendations," p. 4.

42. CDC, "Update: Transmission of HIV Infection," pp. 377–81.

43. Kantrowitz, "Doctors with AIDS," p. 49.

44. "Quayle Pushes AIDS Tests for Doctors," *Washington Times,* June 25, 1991, p. 1, reprinted in the *Congressional Record,* July 11, 1991, p. S9782.

45. Reported by the *Raleigh News and Observer,* June 28, 30, and July 1–3, 1991.

These reports were reprinted in the *Congressional Record,* July 11, 1991, pp. S9780–81.

46. Kantrowitz, "Doctors with AIDS," pp. 48–57.

47. Kantrowitz, "Doctors with AIDS," p. 52.

48. Kantrowitz, "Doctors with AIDS," p. 51.

49. J. W. Cavender, "AIDS in the Health Care Setting: The Congressional Response to the Kimberly Bergalis Case," *Georgia Law Review 26* (Winter 1992), pp. 539–99; and T. E. Margolis, "Health Care Workers and AIDS: HIV Transmission in the Health Care Environment," *Journal of Legal Medicine 13* (Sept. 1992), pp. 357–96.

50. Quote from Bayer, *Private Acts, Social Consequences,* p. 142.

51. *Congressional Record,* July 11, 1991, p. S9782.

52. Sternberg, notes, July 17, 1991.

53. Runnells, *AIDS in the Dental Office?,* p. 183.

54. *Congressional Record,* July 11, 1991, p. S9778.

55. *Congressional Record,* July 18, 1991, p. S10334.

56. J. Monk, "Senator Helms: Force Doctors to Reveal Own HIV Infection," *Charlotte Observer,* July 12, 1991; reprinted in *Congressional Record,* July 18, 1991, p. S10335.

57. Sternberg, "Conservatives Set the Tone," p. A13.

58. *Congressional Record,* July 15, 1991, p. S9977.

59. L. K. Altman, "U.S. Would Curtail Doctors with AIDS," *New York Times,* July 16, 1991, pp. A1, B2.

60. *Congressional Record,* July 18, 1991, p. S10348. Barnes, Rango, Burke, and Chiarello, "The HIV-Infected Health Care Professional," p. 325, fn. 25.

61. DeConcini speaking on ABC, *World News Tonight with Peter Jennings,* July 18, 1991.

62. M. A. Peterson, personal correspondence with author, Oct. 13, 1996.

63. Subcommittee on the Environment, Committee on Energy and Commerce, U.S. House of Representatives, *Prevention of HIV Transmission,* Hearings, 102nd Congress, 1st session, Sept. 19, 26, 1991.

64. Waxman, in Subcommittee on the Environment, Committee on Energy and Commerce, U.S. House of Representatives, *Prevention of HIV Transmission,* pp. 1–2.

65. Dannemeyer, in Subcommittee on the Environment, Committee on Energy and Commerce, U.S. House of Representatives, *Prevention of HIV Transmission,* p. 2.

66. "Statement of C. Everett Koop, Former Surgeon General," in Subcommittee on the Environment, Committee on Energy and Commerce, U.S. House of Representatives, *Prevention of HIV Transmission,* pp. 53–57; P. Hilts,

"Mandatory AIDS Tests for Doctors Would Be Useless," *New York Times*, Sept. 20, 1991, p. A22.

67. Statement of K. Bergalis, in Subcommittee on the Environment, Committee on Energy and Commerce, U.S. House of Representatives, *Prevention of HIV Transmission*, p. 128.

68. Statement of G. Bergalis, in Subcommittee on the Environment, Committee on Energy and Commerce, U.S. House of Representatives, *Prevention of HIV Transmission*, pp. 129–30.

69. G. Bergalis, quoted in Runnells, *AIDS in the Dental Office?*, p. 186.

70. A. Bergalis, quoted in Runnells, *AIDS in the Dental Office?*, p. 186.

71. Runnells, *AIDS in the Dental Office?*, pp. 186–87.

72. D. Ricks, "HRS Official Pins 'Hysteria' on Bergalis," *Orlando Sentinel Tribune*, Sept. 27, 1991, p. A5.

73. G. Ifill, "Congress Kills Penalties in AIDS Disclosure Plan," *New York Times*, Sept. 28, 1991, p. A7.

74. Ifill, "Congress Kills Penalties," p. A7.

75. Ifill, "Congress Kills Penalties," p. A7.

76. W. T. Gormley Jr., "Regulatory Issue Networks in a Federal System," *Polity* 18 (Summer 1986), pp. 595–620.

77. *Congressional Record*, July 18, 1991, p. S10341.

78. CDC, 1991 recommendations, p. 4.

79. CDC, 1991 recommendations, p. 4.

80. CDC, 1991 recommendations, p. 5.

81. CDC, "Open Meeting to Discuss Invasive Procedures Under Consideration for Designation as Exposure-Prone or Not Exposure-Prone" (Atlanta: CDC, Nov. 4, 1991).

82. M. Gladwell, "Medical Groups Reject Limits on HIV-Infected Workers," *Washington Post*, Nov. 5, 1991, p. A1.

83. CDC, "Open Meeting to Discuss Invasive Procedures," p. 78.

84. CDC, "Open Meeting to Discuss Invasive Procedures," p. 45.

85. CDC, "Open Meeting to Discuss Invasive Procedures," p. 38.

86. Altman, "U.S. to Let States Set Rules on AIDS-Infected Health Workers," *New York Times*, June 16, 1992, p. C7.

87. W. Leary, "AMA Backs Off on an AIDS Risk List," *New York Times*, Dec. 15, 1991, p. A38.

88. Gladwell, "Medical Groups Reject Limits," p. A1.

89. M. Cimons, "Plans to Ease Curbs on AIDS-Infected Doctors Is Scrapped," *Los Angeles Times*, June 14, 1992, p. A13.

90. R. T. Craig and L. L. Bryant, "HIV-Infected Health Workers: Debating the Issues," *NCSL State Legislative Report 17* (Aug. 1992), p. 3.

91. Cimons, "Plan to Ease Curbs on AIDS-Infected Doctors Is Scrapped."
92. W. L. Roper, letter to state health officers, June 18, 1992.
93. "States Asked to Decide AIDS Risk," *Philadelphia Inquirer* (June 17, 1992), p. A2.

Chapter Seven

1. AIDS Policy Center, "A Summary of HIV/AIDS Laws from the 1992 State Legislative Sessions" (Washington, D.C.: AIDS Policy Center, Jan. 1993), p. 20ff.
2. F. Shen, "Shaefer Weighs Mandatory AIDS Testing: Governor May Push Legislation Aimed at Health Care Providers," *Washington Post*, Aug. 7, 1991, p. D5.
3. J. C. Van Gieson, D. O'Neal, and D. Salamone, "What's On the Agenda in Tallahassee?" *Orlando Sentinel Tribune*, Jan. 31, 1993, p. G6; L. Bowleg, "Yesterday's News?: Revisiting the Issue of HIV-Infected Patients, Providers," *Intergovernmental AIDS Reports 6* (March 1993), pp. 1–3.
4. Craig and Bryant, "HIV-Infected Health Workers," pp. 3–4.
5. See S. Burris, "HIV-Infected Health Care Workers: The Restoration of Professional Authority," *Archives of Family Medicine 5* (Feb. 1996), pp. 102–106.
6. Barnes, Rango, Burke, and Chiarello, "The HIV-Infected Health Care Professional," pp. 311–30; especially pp. 315–16.
7. *Doe* v. *Westchester County Medical Center*, nos. 1B-E-D–86–116054 and 1B-P-D–87–117683, slip op. (N.Y. State Division of Human Rights, Dec. 12, 1990); reprinted in *New York Law Journal*, Dec. 26, 1990, p. 30.
8. Testimony of G. Wormser, M.D., *Doe* v. *Westchester County Medical Center*, transcript p. 1724–5 (N.Y. State Division of Human Rights, May 19, 1988); cited by Barnes, Rango, Burke, and Chiarello, "The HIV-Infected Health Care Professional," p. 327, fn. 61.
9. N.Y. Public Health Law 2786 (1) (1990).
10. *New York Compendium of Codes, Rules, and Regulations*, title 10, 63.9 (1989); cited by Barnes, Rango, Burke, and Chiarello, "The HIV-Infected Health Care Professional," p. 316, fn. 64.
11. New York State Department of Health, *Policy Statement and Guidelines: Health Care Facilities and HIV-Infected Medical Personnel*, Jan. 18, 1991; reported in L. K. Altman, "New York Won't Tell Doctors with AIDS to Inform Patients," *New York Times*, Jan. 19, 1991, p. A1.
12. C. Gorman, "When Your Doctor Has AIDS: Bucking an Emotional National Crusade, New York Decides Not to Force Physicians to Tell Their Patients," *Time*, Oct. 21, 1991, p. 83.

13. A. Bass, "Health Chief: AIDS Shouldn't Bar Doctors," *Boston Globe*, Oct. 12, 1991, p. 25.

14. *McBarnette v. Feldman*. This case is described in AIDS Policy Center, *Intergovernmental AIDS Reports 5* (Feb. 1992), p. 11.

15. AIDS Policy Center, "State Bills Related to HIV Infected Health Care Providers," *Intergovernmental AIDS Reports* (1992).

16. L. Bowleg, "Yesterday's News?," *Intergovernmental AIDS Reports 6* (Feb. 1993), p. 2.

17. The Illinois Sexually Transmissible Disease Control Act, *Illinois Review of Statutes*, chapter 111½, par. 7401, as amended by P.A. 87–763, effective Oct. 4, 1991.

18. AIDS Policy Center, "A Summary of HIV/AIDS Laws."

19. AIDS Policy Center, "A Summary of HIV/AIDS Laws."

20. H. S. Leeds, "State Spending for HIV/AIDS Education and Training for Health Care Workers," *Intergovernmental AIDS Reports 6* (March 1993), pp. 4–5.

21. AIDS Policy Center, "From Our Files," *Intergovernmental AIDS Reports 6* (March 1993), p. 7.

22. Department of Labor, Occupational Safety and Health Administration, "Occupational Exposure to Bloodborne Pathogens," 29 CFR Part 1910.1030 (Dec. 6, 1991).

23. CDC, "Update: Human Immunodeficiency Virus Infections in Health-Care Workers Exposed to Blood of Infected Patients," *MMWR 36* (May 22, 1987), pp. 285–89.

24. *Congressional Record*, Sept. 11, 1991, p. S12728.

25. OSHA, "Occupational Exposure to Bloodborne Pathogens." Sect. II.

26. *Industrial Union Department, AFL-CIO v. American Petroleum Institute*, 448 U.S. 601, 64 L. Ed. 2d 1010, 100 S. Ct. 2844 (1980), cited in OSHA, "Occupational Exposure to Bloodborne Pathogens."

27. OSHA, "Occupational Exposure to Bloodborne Pathogens." Sect. II.

28. *American Textile Manufacture's Institute, Inc. v. Donovan*, 452 U.S. 490 (1981); cited in OSHA, "Occupational Exposure to Bloodborne Pathogens."

29. *Industrial Union Department, AFL-CIO v. American Petroleum Institute*, 448 U.S. 601, 64 L. Ed. 2d 1010, 100 S. Ct. 2844 (1980), p. 655, 656, n. 62; cited in OSHA, "Occupational Exposure to Bloodborne Pathogens."

30. Statement by Department of Labor assistant secretary Pendergrass, *Congressional Record*, Sept. 11, 1991, p. S12729.

31. OSHA, "Occupational Exposure to Bloodborne Pathogens."

32. 54 *Federal Register* 23042.

33. "AIDS, OSHA Closes Agency's Most Extensive Record, Will Publish Rule Within a Year," *Daily Report for Executives* (May 25, 1990), p. A6.

34. *Congressional Record,* Sept. 11, 1991, p. S12728.

35. *Congressional Record,* Sept. 11, 1991, p. S12726.

36. *Congressional Record,* Sept. 11, 1991, p. S12730.

37. *Congressional Record,* Sept. 11, 1991, p. S12727.

38. For a brief description, see M. F. Goldsmith, "OSHA Bloodborne Pathogens Standard Aims to Limit Occupational Transmission," *JAMA 267* (June 3, 1992), pp. 2853–54.

39. See, for example, S. Kelman, *Regulating America, Regulating Sweden: A Comparative Study of Occupational Safety and Health Policy* (Cambridge, Mass.: MIT Press, 1981).

40. *American Dental Association and Home Health Services and Staffing Association, Inc., v. Lynn Martin, Secretary of Labor, and OSHA, U.S. Department of Labor,* Nos. 1 91–3865, 92–1482, U.S. Court of Appeals, 7th Circuit (Jan. 28, 1993).

41. *ADA v. Martin,* p. 825.

42. *ADA v. Martin,* p. 825.

43. *ADA v. Martin,* p. 825.

44. *ADA v. Martin,* pp. 825, 829.

45. See C. R. Sunstein, *After the Rights Revolution: Reconceiving the Regulatory State* (Cambridge, Mass.: Harvard University Press, 1990), pp. 239–42.

46. For an application of this logic, see *Competitive Enterprise Institute* v. the *National Highway Traffic Safety Administration (NHTSA),* 294 U.S. App. D.C. 35, 956 F.2d 321 (D.C. Cir. 1992).

47. *ADA v. Martin,* p. 838.

48. *ADA v. Martin,* pp. 839, 840.

49. See R. Marcus and others, "Transmission of Human Immunodeficiency Virus (HIV) in Healthcare Settings Worldwide," *Bulletin of the World Health Organization 67* (1989), pp. 577–82.

50. *ADA v. Martin,* pp. 831–32.

51. *ADA v. Martin,* p. 843.

52. *Gade* v. *National Solid Wastes Management Ass'n,* 120 L. Ed. 2d 73, 112 S. Ct. 2374 (1992).

53. See T. B. Metzloff, "Researching Litigation: The Medical Malpractice Example," *Law and Contemporary Problems 51* (1988), pp. 199–242.

54. See R. A. Kagan, "Adversarial Legalism and American Government," *Journal of Public Policy Analysis and Management 10* (1991), pp. 369–406.

55. For a discussion of the legal cases, see Burris, "HIV-Infected Health Care Workers"; E. Gautier, *The Legal Rights and Obligations of HIV-Infected Health Care Workers* (American Association of Physicians for Human Rights, San Francisco, and National Lawyers Guild, New York, 1993).

56. *Hofman* v. *Blackmon,* 241 So.2d 752 (Fla. 4th DCA 1970). R. Montgomery,

"Kimberly Bergalis: Professional Malpractice and AIDS," unpublished manuscript, Sept. 7, 1995, p. 17.

57. Montgomery, "Kimberly Bergalis." See also *Driskill* v. *CIGNA Dental Health of Florida, Inc.,* no. 91–177, 19th Jud. Cir., Martin County, Fla. (1991,) cited by A. S. Oddi, "Reverse Informed Consent," pp. 1417–76.

58. Montgomery, "Kimberly Bergalis," p. 16.

59. See Montgomery, "Kimberly Bergalis," pp. 19, 21.

60. 543 So.2d 209, Fla. 1989.

61. 781 S.W.2d 58, Mo. 1989.

62. C. Woolsey, "Insurers Face Claims by Patient of Dentist Who Contracted AIDS," *Business Insurance,* Feb. 25, 1991, p. 22.

63. Patient report by P. B. Toon, M.D., Nov. 28, 1990.

64. Palca, "CDC Closes the Case of the Florida Dentist," pp. 1130–31.

65. Barr, "In Defense of the AIDS Dentist," p. 80.

66. L. G. Abele and R. W. DeBry, "Florida Dental Case: Research Affiliation and Ethics," letter to *Science 21* (Feb. 1992), p. 903.

67. Palca, "The Case of the Florida Dentist," pp. 392–94.

68. R. W. DeBry and others, "Dental HIV Transmission," p. 691.

69. Ou and others, "Molecular Epidemiology," pp. 1165–71.

70. See D. M. Hillis, J. P. Huelsenbeck, and C. W. Cunningham, "Application and Accuracy of Molecular Phylogenies," *Science 264* (Apr. 29, 1994), pp. 671–76; and Hillis and J. P. Huelsenbeck, "Support for Dental HIV Transmission," pp. 24–25.

71. DeBry and others, "Dental HIV Transmission," p. 691.

72. Barr, "In Defense of the AIDS Dentist," p. 68.

73. Barr, "In Defense of the AIDS Dentist," p. 69.

74. See, for example, "Lawsuits Blamed on 'Unsound' Policy for HIV-Positive Health Care Workers," *AIDS Alert 9* (March 1994), p. 33.

75. Burris, "HIV-Infected Health Care Workers."

76. *Faya* v. *Almaraz,* 329 Md. 435, 620 A.2d 327 (1993); *Marchica* v. *Long Island Rail Road,* 31 F.3d 1197 (2d Cir. 1994), cert. denied, 115 S. Ct. 727 (1995).

77. For cases in which the plaintiff had to prove physical contact, Burris cites *Poole* v. *Alpha Therapeutic Corporation,* 698 F.Supp. 1367 (N.D.Ill.1988); *Taylor* v. *Morrison Dental Associates, P.C.,* No. X91–2445–H (Ga. Super. Apr. 21, 1994), in *AIDS Litigation Report,* 28 June 1994, 12081–12094; *Barrett* v. *Danbury Hospital,* 232 Conn. 22, 654 A.2d 748 (1995); and *K.A.C.* v. *Benson,* 527 N.W. 2d 553 (Minn. 1995). For cases in which the plaintiff had to prove "actual exposure," Burris cites *Johnson* v. *West Virginia University Hospitals,* 186 W.Va. 648, 413 S.E.2d 889 (W.Va. 1991); *Funeral Service by Gregory, Inc.* v. *Bluefield Community Hospital,* 186 W.Va. 424, 413 S.E.2d 79

(1991); *Carroll* v. *The Sisters of Saint Francis Health Services, Inc.,* 868 S.W.d 585 (Tn. Super. 1993); *Burk* v. *Sage Products, Inc.,* 747 F.Supp. 285 (E.D.Pa. 1990); *Doe* v. *Surgicare of Joliet, Inc.,* 643 N.E. 2d 1200 (Ill.App.), appeal denied, 158 Ill. 2d 568 (1994); *Lubowitz* v. *Albert Einstein Medical Center,* 424 Pa.Super. 468, 623 A.2d 3 (1993); *Hare* v. *State,* 570 N.Y.S. 2d 125 (App. Div.), appeal denied, 575 N.Y.S.2d 455 (1991); *Brzoska* v. *Olsen,* 1994 Del. Super. LEXIS 230 (May 2, 1994); *Kerins* v. *Hartley,* 27 Cal.App.4th 1062, 33 Cal.Rptr.2d 172 (1994); *Ordway* v. *County of Suffolk,* 154 Misc. 2d 269, 583 N.Y.S.2d 1014 (Sup. Ct. 1992) (requiring objective facts regarding exposure and medical consequences as "guarantee of genuineness"); see Burris, "HIV-Infected Health Care Workers."

78. *K.A.C.* v. *Benson,* 527 N.W.2d 553 (Minn. 1995) and *Canterbury* v. *Spence,* 464 F.2d 772 (D.C. Cir. 1972).

79. This was the situation in *Taylor* v. *Morrison Dental Associates, P.C.,* No. X91–2445–H (Ga. Super. April 21, 1994) in *AIDS Litigation Reporter* (June 28, 1994), pp. 12081–94; *Kerins* v. *Hartley,* 27 Cal. App. 4th 1062, 33 Cal.Rptr.2d 172 (1994); cited by Burris, "HIV-Infected Health Care Workers."

80. Kantrowitz, "Doctors with AIDS," p. 51.

81. "Lawsuits Blamed on 'Unsound' Policy for HIV-Positive Health Care Workers," p. 33.

82. *K.A.C.* v. *Benson,* 527 N.W.2d 553 (Minnesota 1995).

83. Burris, "HIV-Infected Health Care Workers," p. 104.

84. See D. Beasley, "Courts," *Atlanta Journal & Constitution,* June 14, 1992, p. D6; *Johnson* v. *West Virginia University Hospitals,* 186 W. Va. 648, 413 S.E.2d 889 (1991).

85. S. D. Watson, "Eliminating Fear Through Comparative Risk: Docs, AIDS, and the Antidiscrimination Ideal," *Buffalo Law Review 40* (1992), pp. 739–807; and Barnes, Rango, Burke, and Chiarello, "The HIV-Infected Health Care Professional," p. 18.

86. *Doe* v. *District of Columbia,* 796 F. Supp. 559, 569 (D.D.C. 1992); *Doe* v. *Attorney General,* 1995 U.S. App. LEXIS 16264 (9th Cir. June 30, 1995); re Westchester County Medical Center, 2. Emp. Prac. Guide (CCH) para 5340 at 6999–323 to 324 (April 20, 1992); Health Care Daily, "Hospital to Reinstate HIV Positive Nurse to a Clinical Care Position," *Health Law Reporter 1* (Jan. 5, 1993), pp. 411; cited in Burris, "HIV-Infected Health Care Workers."

87. *Leckelt* v. *Board of Commissioners,* 909 F.2d 820, 829 (5th Cir. 1990); *Estate of Behringer* v. *The Medical Center at Princeton,* 592 A.2d 1251 (N.J. Super 1991); *Bradley* v. *University of Texas,* 3 F.3d 922 (5th Cir. 1993), cert denied 114 S. Ct. 1071 (1994); *Doe* v. *Washington University,* 780 F. Supp. 628, 634

(E.D. Mo. 1991); *Doe v. University of Maryland Medical System Corporation.*, 50 F.3d 1261 (4th Cir. 1995); *Mauro v. Borgess Medical Center*, 1995 U.S. Dist. LEXIS 6910 (W.D. Mich. May 4, 1995); cited by Burris in "HIV-Infected Health Care Workers."

88. *Doe v. Mercy Health Corp. of Southeastern Pennsylvania*, DC Epa, No. 92–6711, described in "HIV-Infected Doctor Charges Hospital Restrictions Illegally Discriminate," *BNA Health Care Daily*, Dec. 24, 1992.

89. R. Black, "Infected Surgeon's Suit May Test HIV Policy," *Dallas Morning News*, Feb. 18, 1993, p. 33A.

90. "HIV-Infected Doctor Charges Hospital Restrictions Illegally Discriminate," *AIDS Alert 9* (Mar. 1994), p. 33.

91. "Lawsuits Blamed on 'Unsound' Policy for HIV-Positive Health Care Workers," p. 33.

92. Interview with Burris, Jan. 29, 1996.

93. *Boulais v. Lustig*, No. BC038105, Cal. Super. Ct. (1993). The surgical technician was awarded $102,500.

94. See T. Pristin, "Nurse Cut by Scalpel Names HIV-Positive Patient, Who Countersues," *Los Angeles Times*, Oct. 30, 1991, p. B3; P. Hager, "High Court Lets AIDS Patient Continue Privacy Invasion Suit," *Los Angeles Times*, Jan. 10, 1992, p. A27.

Chapter Eight

1. Cox New Service, "Feeling the Fury of the Bergalis Case: HRS Officials Say They Were Unfair Targets of Angry Letter," *Orlando Sentinel Tribune*, Aug. 21, 1991, p. A1.

2. Rom, *Public Spirit in the Thrift Tragedy.*

3. Panem, *The AIDS Bureaucracy*, pp. 31–35. For more details about this dispute (including letters exchanged between Congressman Weiss and CDC Director Foege), see U.S. House of Representatives, Oversight Committee on Government Operations, "Federal Response to AIDS," hearings, Aug. 1–2, 1983.

4. "GAO Review of Dental Case Supports CDC Conclusions," *AIDS Alert 7* (Dec. 1992), pp. 183–85; quote on p. 183.

5. GAO, *AIDS: CDC's Investigation*, p. 2.

6. Panem, *The AIDS Bureaucracy*, pp. 138–41.

7. Letter from B. Schatz and N. Offen, GLMA, to H. Gayle, director, National Center on HIV, STD, TB, and Prevention, June 26, 1996, pp. 1, 3.

8. K. Bergalis, "I Blame Every One of You Bastards."

9. For a theoretical development of the institutional preferences of interests facing uncertainty, see T. Moe, "The Politics of Bureaucratic Structure," in J. Chubb and P. E. Peterson, eds., *Can the Government Govern?* (Washington, D.C.: Brookings Institution, 1990).

10. S. Burris, "Public Health, AIDS Exceptionalism, and the Law," *John Marshall Law Review 27* (Winter 1994), p. 260.

11. See especially L. J. Marcus and others, *Renegotiating Health Care: Resolving Conflict to Build Collaboration* (San Francisco: Jossey-Bass, 1995); L. Susskind and P. Field, *Dealing with an Angry Public: The Mutual Gains Approach to Resolving Disputes* (New York: Free Press, 1996).

12. Marcus and others, *Renegotiating Health Care,* p. 37.

13. See for example P. A. Marshall and others, "Patients' Fear of Contracting the Acquired Immunodeficiency Syndrome from Physicians," *Archives of Internal Medicine 150* (July 1990), pp. 1501–6.

14. See L. Gostin, "Hospitals, Health Care Professionals, and AIDS: The 'Right to Know' the Health Status of Professionals and Patients," *Maryland Law Review 48* (1992), p. 12.

15. Runnells, *AIDS in the Dental Office?,* p. 34.

16. Runnells, *AIDS in the Dental Office?,* p. 35.

17. D. Moss, "AIDS Shatters Teen's World," *USA Today,* May 13, 1993, p. 3A.

18. The idea of the "veil of ignorance" is developed in great subtlety and detail by J. Rawls in *A Theory of Justice* (Cambridge, Mass.: Harvard University Press, 1980).

19. *Cruzan* v. *Director, Missouri Department of Health,* 110 S.Ct. 2841 (1990), quoting from *Union Pacific Railroad* v. *Botsford,* 141 U.S. 250, 251 (1891); cited by K. C. Lieberman and A. R. Derse, "HIV-Positive Health Care Workers and the Obligation to Disclose: Do Patients Have a Right to Know?," *Journal of Legal Medicine 13* (1992), pp. 333–56; quote on p. 342.

20. J. Gray, "Why Bad Doctors Aren't Kicked Out of Medicine," *Medical Economics,* Jan. 20, 1992, pp. 126–49.

About the Author

Mark Carl Rom is assistant professor of government and public policy at Georgetown University and Robert Wood Johnson Scholar in health policy research at the University of California, Berkeley. He is the author of *Public Spirit in the Thrift Tragedy* and coauthor with Paul E. Peterson of *Welfare Magnets: A New Case for a National Welfare Standard*. Rom also served as the principal investigator of the study *AIDS: CDC's Investigation of HIV Transmissions by a Dentist* for the U.S. General Accounting Office.

～～ Index

A

ABC, 4

Abele, L., 148–149

Acer, D.: AIDS condition of, while in practice, 82–83; AIDS nondisclosure by, 97–98; authorization for release of patient names of, 42; blood samples taken from, 28, 29, 53; CDC interview with, 27–29, 75, 82, 90; CDC interview with, critique of, 28–29; CDC interview with, report of, 179–180; childhood and life history of, 86–87; competence of, 83–84; dental practice of, 28, 74–78; family relationships of, 87–88; HIV virus of, genetic analysis of, 52, 58–61; and homicide transmission theory, 84–90; legal counsel to, 28, 42; letter of, to patients, 43–44, 52; personality of, 85–88, 91; and political terrorist theory, 88–89; retirement of, 28; and sexual transmission theory, 71–72; as source of Bergalis' infection, CDC announcement of, 36–41; as source of other patients' infection, 2–3, 41–48; transmission method of, theories of, 71–92. *See also* Florida dentist case

Acer, H. (mother), 74

Acer, K. (brother), 88

Acer clinic, 74–78; infection control practices of, 75–78; staff of, 75, 76–77

Acer patients: contact of, with Acer

authorization, 41–42; contact of, with Acer letter, 43–48; and contaminated equipment theory, 78–80; in control group, 64; and direct blood contact theory, 82–83; gender and age of, 88; and genetic sequencing study, 52–53, 60–61, 68–69; with HIV, field investigation of, 45–48; with HIV, infected by Acer, 2; with HIV, number of, 2–3, 45; HIV testing of, 44–45; and homicide theory, 88, 89; invasive procedures performed on, 83; theory of "mystery," 80. *See also* Bergalis, K.; Driskill, R.; Johnson, S.; Patient D; Patient F; Patient H; Patient J; Shoemaker, L.; Webb, B.; Yecs, J.

ACT-UP, 89

Administrative Procedures Act (APA), 114, 139

AIDS: and blood banks, 8–9; history of, and CDC, 7–10

AIDS Bureaucracy, The (Panem), 162

AIDS Policy Center survey, 137

AIDS reporting, 16–20; in Florida, 16, 25–26; and HIV tracing challenges, 20–23; legal authority for, 16; progression of, in Bergalis case, 25–27; and risk factor identification, 17–20; and "reportable" disease classification, 16; timing of, 25–27

AIDS Research and Information Act, 138, 139–140

Alcohol sterilization, 75

Alienation, 86–87